PRAISE FOR *The Dragon with F*

Deborah Miller is not only a highly trained professional, she is a gifted healer that has a special gift for helping parents and children dealing with cancer. What Deborah teaches gives them the hope and tools they need for healing. I recommend this book to anyone dealing with a challenging illness, child or adult. You will benefit greatly by her teachings.
— Carol Tuttle, best selling author of *The Child Whisperer*

This book is a distillation of love and affection, and dedication not only to a spectacular Technique, but also to children and their serious illnesses. I heartily recommend that if you are into Tapping, you need to read this book with all your heart. There is so much yet to learn in this amazing adventure called EFT.
— Till Schilling, Emocional Training Ecuador

Ever since hearing of her great work, Deborah Miller has been a hero of mine. I'm very happy that she's come out with a book so that this healing work can be experienced by a much larger audience. So many great examples of tapping to follow along with, beautifully illustrated – this book is a wonderful gift for children (of all ages) dealing with illness… and the people who love them.
— Brad Yates, Author of *The Wizard's Wish*

A beautiful book that will help parents, children and caregivers discover relief in the midst of a difficult time. By teaching tapping, Deborah empowers you with a tool that can help you every step of the way.
— Jessica Ortner, Producer of The Tapping Solution
www.TheTappingSolution.com

This little book will be an incredible gift for children all over the world who are confronting the rigors of cancer (or other serious illnesses), as well as for their parents. It distills Dr. Miller's [Dr. Miller's degree is in Cell and Molecular Biology] compassionate and effective work with hundreds of children into a simple, do-it-yourself resource that will give parents a remarkably effective tool for helping their child cope and thrive with the psychological challenges of cancer and its treatment."
— David Feinstein, Ph.D.
Author, *Energy Psychology Interactive*

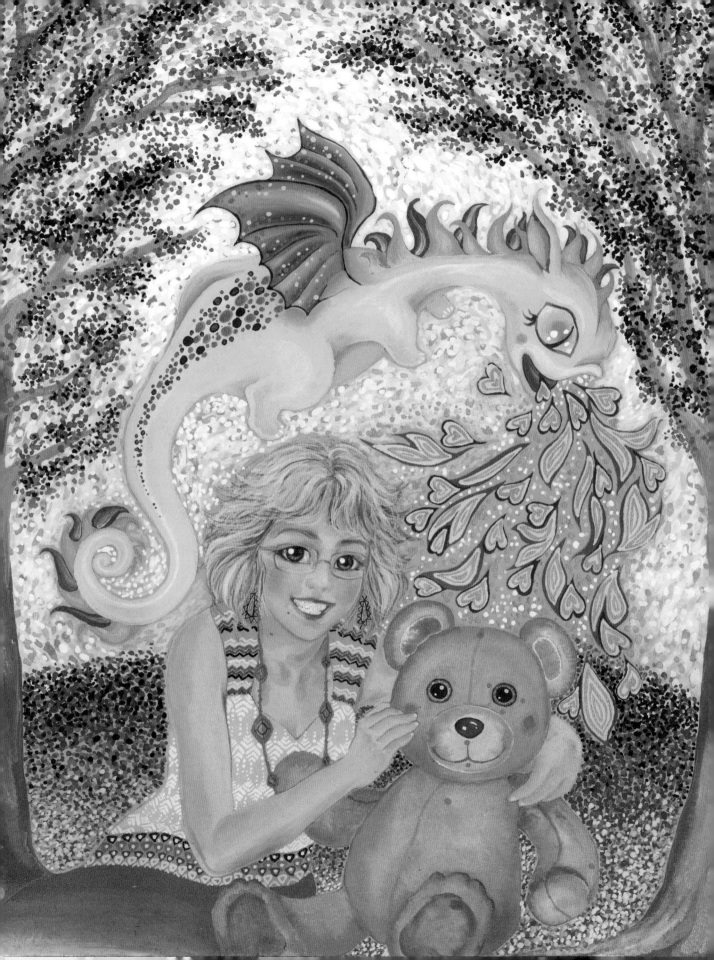

PRAISE FOR *The Dragon with Flames of Love*

Deborah's work has been recognized internationally by many in the healing arts community and with the introduction of this book luckily many more will reap the rewards of her wisdom from her dedication and wisdom in the field. This book is a fantastic resource for anyone dealing with pediatric cancer or any other life-threatening illness for that matter. The examples, techniques, and explanation of how EFT works serve to inspire and educate all who are invested in helping children and their families.

– Alina Frank, EFT trainer

My dear friend Deborah's courageous work is leading edge, from the heart and powerful. Her book, "The Dragon With Flames of Love" is a must read for all families going through the challenge of children facing serious illnesses. Relief, peace and healing can begin as soon as you start reading and Tapping.

– Lori Leyden, Ph.D.
Founder of Create Global Healing
Head of The Tapping Solution Foundation

"The Dragon with Flames of Love" is an invaluable tool for parents of children who are facing serious health issues. It presents usable tools in a straightforward and loving way. I love the way it empowers both parents and children to respond to the struggles they are facing in a way that puts them in control. Deborah's experience and compassion comes through so clearly in this easy to use book.

– Gene Monterastelli
Editor TappingQandA.com

Deborah Miller's book, "The Dragon with Flames of Love," is an act of love. Each page of this book is an invitation to trust in human beings, each story is an opportunity to rediscover the excitement, each feeling put into it is an investment in consciousness. With EFT as a shield and defense, the dragon as an ally and companion, and with Deborah in her role as vital sorceress, these stories, this book, these pages, are a gentle wind that provides a light breeze of confidence in human beings and of love for life. Get close to this dragon to discover the warmth of these flames that are now being lit and that after reading this book, you will not want to extinguish either.

– Luis Bueno, Coach, EFT Trainer, Ericksonian Hypnosis Expert
www.efeteando.com

What a beautiful and important book! Deborah Miller has been doing incredible work with children with cancer for years, now her wisdom, love and powerful experiences are available for the world to learn from. I highly suggest you read this book today.

– Nick Ortner, Author of *The Tapping Solution*

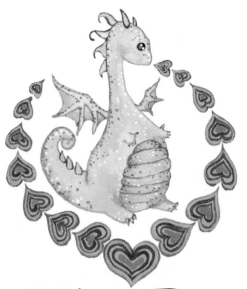

The Dragon *with* Flames *of* Love

Helping Children
with Serious Illness
Improve the Quality
of Their Lives

Deborah D. Miller, Ph.D.

ISBN: 978-0-9763200-6-7

Illustrations by: Alexandra Gapihan, http://www.alexandragapihan.com,
https://www.facebook.com/pages/Moon-Risce-Estudio/176208062409431
Copy Edited by: Deborah-Miriam Leff, PickyPickyPicky.net
Graphic Design by: Deborah Perdue, www.illuminationgraphics.com

Further information:
www.OaxacaProject.com
www.FindTheLightWithin.com
ddmiller7@FindTheLightWithin.com

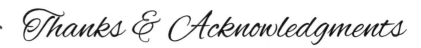

Thanks & Acknowledgments

I'd like to express my gratitude to the following people:

My parents, Eldor and Ida Miller, for raising me on a farm in North Dakota, which gave me a deep love and respect for all living beings, and for leading me to the path of complementary therapy when I was a teenager.

Vera Malbaski for translating these stories into Spanish with such detail and attention to the wording, and for her enduring friendship.

Till Schilling for being an extraordinary friend and supporter, as well as the creator of TappyBear, who has played a major role in my work with children with cancer.

Alexandra Gapihan for creating with such love and attention these magnificent illustrations based on the children I've worked with and for her beautiful use of color, texture and imagination to make the presentation of this information enchanting for children and adults alike.

Sara Roberts for doing a beautiful job of editing the Spanish language version of this book, using her insights and attention to detail in order to make the text clear, concise and flow easily.

Deborah-Miriam Leff for her friendship, and editing the English language version of this book with her keen eye and ability to perfect the final presentation of the information.

Deborah Perdue for creating the attractive graphic design for the book that compliments and shows off the content and illustrations in a way that makes the book a delight to look at and fun to read.

Ana Maria, Adriana A., Jennifer, Adriana F., Kathilyn, Emilio and all those who have supported me in my efforts to create this book.

Maribel Martínez Ruiz for her financial support for the preparation of this book, and her faith in me and this project that compliments her desire to help mothers raise their children in a more loving way.

Dr. Armando Quero Hernández, head oncologist at the Hospital General Aurelio Valdivieso in Oaxaca, Mexico, for his openness to and awareness of the emotional needs of child patients, and for allowing me access to the children, the doctors, nurses and the hospital.

Dr. Karla Gómez Márquez, oncologist, whose steadfast support allows me to continue working with the children, their families and the medical staff.

Irais Pacheco, head nurse, for allowing the nurses to work with me.

The parents of the children for opening their hearts and permitting me to help them and their children.

The children — the bravest, most incredible souls I know — for their beauty, joy and love in the midst of their healing journey, and for how they deeply touch my heart and soul. I will be forever grateful to each and every one of them.

TABLE OF CONTENTS

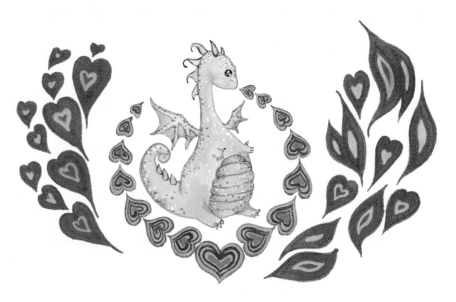

INTRODUCTION

*I*n this book, I explain how I first came to work with children with cancer in a hospital setting. I share my experience, knowledge and my wishes for you as parents and for your children, and describe how the technique of EFT works. This is followed by a description of the effects of EFT on real life children with cancer. ('EFT' and 'Tapping' are the exact same thing, and these terms are used interchangeably throughout this book.)

The book is filled with stories and the actual phrases I used while doing EFT with the children. We used EFT for various typical situations that a child with cancer or a serious illness experiences in the course of treatment — for example, having an IV put in. While Tapping, the child relaxes and the veins tend to come to the surface. This makes it easier to insert an IV. Wouldn't you like your child to be poked with a needle only once instead of three or four times?

You'll find specific information on how to use EFT with your own child within the stories that are based on real-life experiences working with children with cancer. The stories show how this technique helps children feel better and enables them to suffer less, emotionally and physically, and empowers them to participate in their own healing journey.

It is a well-known and generally accepted fact that a major part of recovering from a serious illness is a positive mental attitude, since state of mind directly affects the physiology of the body. Consequently, techniques such as EFT can play a vital role in helping patients – in this case, children – who are recovering from cancer and those whose bodies are beyond recovery. In either case one can reduce emotional and physical suffering, increase comfort, joy, peace and love with EFT, creating the quality of life that every child deserves.

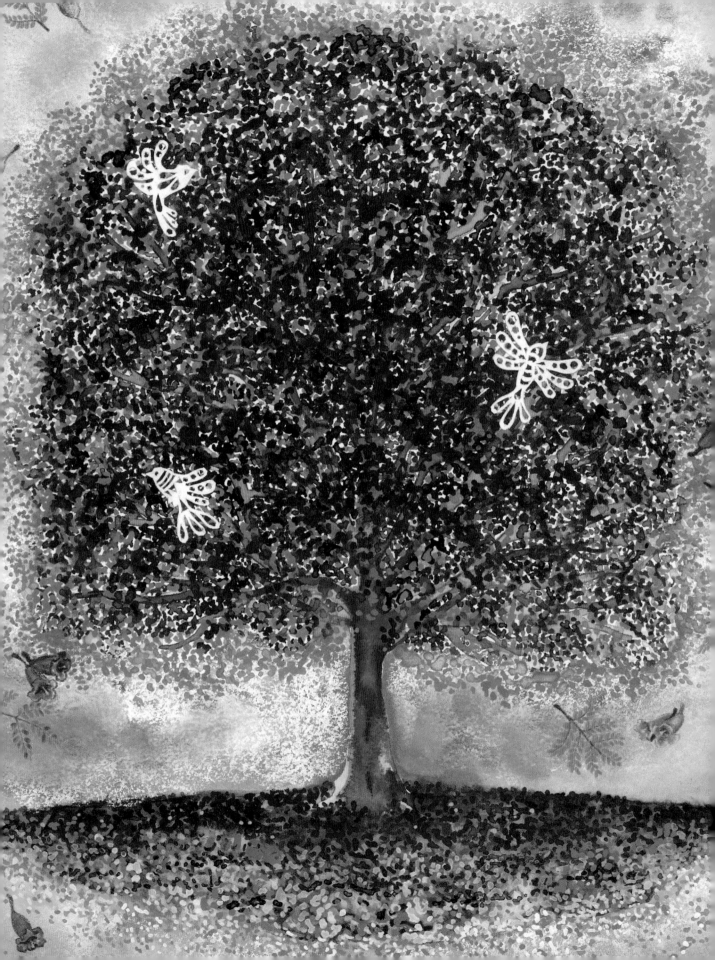

FOREWORD

My deepest desire is for more children with serious illness to feel empowered and able to manage everything they encounter during a journey with an illness. I was given the amazing opportunity to do this when I was invited to work with children with cancer in a hospital setting in September 2007. Since then, and to the present day, I go into the hospital every week, Monday to Friday. At the time of writing, I have worked with some 350 children, from as young as one month through eighteen years old. These children have been dealing with the following types of illnesses: acute and chronic Lymphocytic and Myeloid Leukemias, Lymphomas, Osteosarcomas, Hepatocellular carcinomas; tumors of the brain, stomach, liver, throat, lungs, abdomen, ovaries, testicles, eyes, soft tissues and kidneys; Hodgkin's lymphoma, Wilms' tumor, Ewing's sarcoma, Rhabdomyosarcoma, Hemophilia and Sickle Cell Anemia.

I've assisted these children and their families in dealing with the shocking diagnoses, as well as with the feelings of fear, sadness, anger, frustration, apathy and powerlessness that they experience. I've been helping them release the deeper physical and emotional suffering associated with a serious illness by using specific techniques which allow them to reduce their pain and symptoms and improve their immune systems. I teach the children how to apply Emotional Freedom Technique (EFT or Tapping) to themselves, so that they can reduce their suffering and pain, and, at the same time, improve their ability to be in control of their emotions. One of the greatest benefits of EFT is that it is fast and easy to use. In a very short time – minutes – a child can relax and smile, play or go to sleep calmly. The results have been powerful, empowering and deeply moving to see.

These children, and my experiences with them, have taught me so much. They inspired me to write this book in order to share the knowledge I have acquired with more children and their families around the world. By doing so, my hope is that greater numbers of children with serious illness can learn how to improve the quality of their lives in a powerful, yet gentle and easy, way.

The stories in this book are based on my personal knowledge and experience. They show the skills and techniques used in real-life situations, where I do Tapping with children who are dealing with cancer. My desire is to offer children, parents and family members the tools, as well as the hope, to change their overall experience while dealing with serious illness. It no longer has to be a period of suffering, but can evolve and change towards greater ease, relief and even joy and laughter. It is possible — I have seen it happen.

Techniques such as EFT empower the child and his or her family members, enabling them to make good choices. When we have the tools and knowledge to improve our emotional state, we feel more empowered and at peace. In terms of recovery, there is a positive outcome to this: we improve our ability to focus our body's own power to heal. This inner power may change the whole experience for the better, which in turn can change the outcome.

Giving hope to a child who has a serious illness is one of the greatest gifts we can give. It changes their perspective and their desire to get better, and allows them to be more in control of what they think and feel. All of this is complementary to their medical treatments and can help make those treatments more effective.

You will see how invaluable this program is for children and families in the hospital with *any* illness, not only serious illness such as cancer. In addition to providing you with a tool to help you support your child and your family during time of illness, my heartfelt desire is that this book will inspire you to see how you might assist me in creating more programs like this one in hospitals everywhere. After you have finished reading, and have practiced Tapping, I will share with you the ways you can support this wonderful vision.

May you be inspired to be part of that vision
Namasté,
Deborah

HOW I CAME TO USE EFT ON KIDS WITH CANCER AT THE HOSPITAL

Life takes you in many directions and some lead to the most amazing experiences, such as my journey into the hospital to help children with cancer.

How does one begin such an intense, enormous project as using EFT on kids with cancer, in a hospital of all places? Amazingly enough, it started in the simplest way. I was invited to participate in the Fundraiser for Kids with Cancer in a local park in July of 2007. I had just gotten my new TappyBear – the stuffed bear that has the Tapping points marked on it – and was eager to see how children responded to him. I had worked with children before but never children with cancer, and I wasn't prepared for the sight of the kids in their pale green gowns lying on mats in the park with IVs. I had gone there that day thinking, "Let's see what happens. I'll spend a few hours lending a hand and helping some children feel a little better." That simple idea led to a lifelong project that continues to grow and fill my heart with love.

My experience that day was a delight because of what transpired. We were in a park, with the kids lying on cots under makeshift tents. It is quite striking to see these beautiful children in pale green gowns with little to no hair, some calm, some very weak, some with IVs, some silent, some distant.

I worked with four children that day. The first was Cinthia. She had the roundest face, and even though she did not see well out of one eye, she paid close attention. I can remember that meeting with such clarity, because it touched my heart. I introduced myself and told her TappyBear was my helper and that we had come to help her feel better. She smiled and was open to trying EFT, especially because using TappyBear looked like it would be fun. Doing EFT together made her feel markedly more relaxed and reduced her discomfort. I was glad, as it was such an encouraging start.

With the other children, I had varying success. One of them was open to EFT, while another was still in shock from finding out that she had leukemia. I did find that tapping with her parents brought them some welcome relief. Another child was very shy. Yet, each

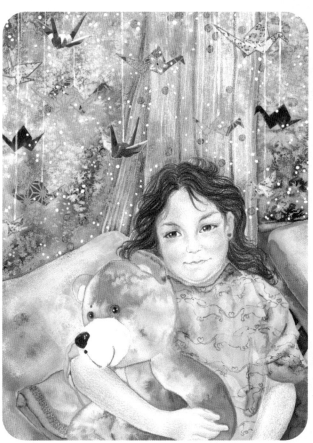

Cinthia – the first child with whom I used EFT and TappyBear in the park.

child relaxed in some way. In each case, TappyBear was a soft and gentle way to approach these children, very different from their experience in the hospital environment with needles and medicines.

After tapping with the children at the fundraiser in the park, I spoke to the doctor in charge of the cancer ward. I commented that it would be interesting to apply EFT in the hospital itself. He agreed. When I went home that day, I wondered why I had suggested this — I had never imagined myself working with children with cancer. But sometimes a deeper heart connection, and one's mission in life, guides one's words, as it did in this case. The idea still had to settle, both for the doctor and myself. It took two months before we managed to reconnect. The day we finally met, September 14, 2007, is a memorable day for me. It was the beginning of a much bigger journey and learning experience in my life.

It started out simply enough, with the doctor and I discussing EFT and the needs of these children beyond the physical treatments they received at the hospital. Because he understood just how much these children and their families needed emotional support, he essentially gave me the freedom to do whatever I could with EFT — and together with my trusty TappyBear, I did so.

I began by demonstrating and teaching EFT to the nursing staff, as they are in immediate contact with the children on a daily basis. I wanted them to know exactly what I was up to, so as not to be surprised by the funny-looking tapping and stuffed bear I would be using, as well as to experience EFT for themselves. I led them through a few rounds of EFT and we ended up laughing, yawning and relaxing. It created a beautiful connection between these nurses, who care so diligently for the children, and I.

Initially, when I met the nurses, I could feel that they were stressed and tired from the amount of work they had in caring for these children, especially since getting too attached to any one of the kids is difficult and has emotional consequences if he or she does not survive. I truly believe that connecting with the nurses has been one of the keys to success, as their support has proved instrumental at the hospital. They freely allow me to work, both with them and with the children.

When I arrived at the Children's Oncology Area in the hospital, much to my surprise, the first girl I saw was Cinthia. She was glad to see me and TappyBear's blue bag on my shoulder. She told me excitedly that she remembered how to tap, had taught her dad how to do it, and they now tapped together. How wonderful that after ten minutes of tapping with me, she could recognize its value, use it and teach someone else how to do it with her. She was the first recipient of a TappyBear, and I knew right away that I would need many more. Thus far, I have been able to give over 150 children with cancer their very own TappyBears. Every time I give a child a TappyBear, I see the other children looking at me with hope in their eyes that they will receive the next one.

INITIAL PERCEPTIONS

When I began, the children's cancer ward had a waiting room, where up to twenty-five parents and children waited for treatments, and it had two rooms with beds. One of them had three beds in it, and the other had six.

The first day I walked into the cancer ward, I was overwhelmed by the feeling of sadness, pain, misery and fear that I sensed, as if I hit a wall of these emotions when I came in. I saw a mother and child huddled together, anxiously, in a corner, and there were about thirty more people in the room in a similar state. I could sense that they each felt alone in their own misery. It was a lonely, isolated and depressing picture that deeply saddened me.

With Cinthia and TappyBear as my ice-breaker, I began to shed my doubts about being able to do Tapping in the hospital and sat down to tap with her, observed by the others. Cinthia's smile was more than enough proof that this was only the beginning.

When I began using EFT, the children and parents who tapped with me began to feel relief on many levels. With time, and as more and more of the children and parents learned EFT, the atmosphere on the ward gradually changed and improved.

NOTICEABLE CHANGES

One morning I walked in and four children with their parents were having breakfast together and laughing. This was so remarkable that even the doctor noticed it and commented about it to me.

On another visit, the children were playing games together or on their own, whereas I'd previously observed a lack of energy or interaction. They were laughing and talking to each other. They were doing puzzles, drawing and coloring. They were playing with a ball and constructing things out of Legos.

Another change was that the parents were talking, sharing experiences and helping each other out. One mother told me that before learning EFT she couldn't help anyone else. She was so absorbed in her problems with her own child, that she was unable to even notice what was going on with the others, much less help them. Now she said she felt empowered, because she felt calm and more relaxed in the face of her child's cancer. In fact, she is currently one of the mothers who goes out of her way to help the other children and parents on the ward.

The next aspect that I was amazed by, was that the nurses became more relaxed as they started to enjoy interacting with children who no longer felt afraid (or felt less afraid) of them and of the treatments they gave them.

A delightful coincidence was that the only place in the whole hospital that got a new paint job was the children's cancer ward. It went from drab gray walls and dark blue doors, to fresh and inviting colors such as a beautiful soft yellow with stuffed animal borders, or light blue walls with scenes from the sea.

The parents themselves show markedly reduced anxiety and a lower intensity of fear, so they can allow themselves to be joyful with their children.

One of the best collective outcomes of using EFT was that the doctor and nurses found increased compliance among the children regarding taking their medications or coming to the hospital for treatments and injections.

The most noticeable change is that now, when I walk into the cancer ward, the energy feels light and comfortable. The constant presence and seriousness of the disease is still there, but not the intense fear of it, nor the inability to manage it. Laughter is now regularly heard coming from the ward.

For me, these changes alone have made it worth bringing the gift of EFT to the hospital.

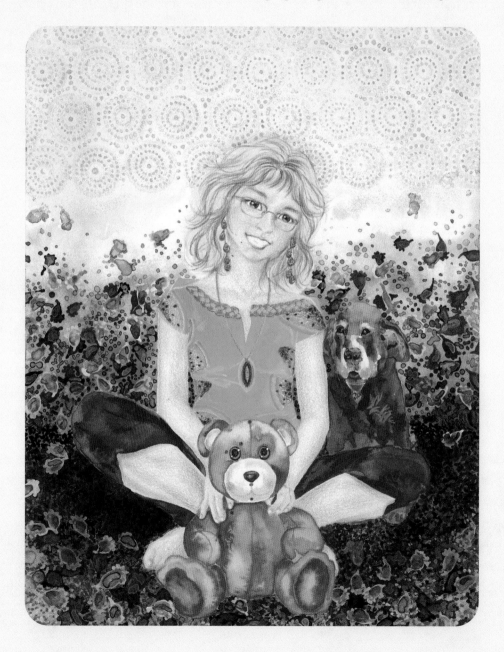

WHAT IS EMOTIONAL FREEDOM TECHNIQUES (EFT) OR TAPPING?

*E*FT or Tapping has been described as "acupuncture for emotions, without the needles." It has its roots in ancient Chinese medicine and the modern science of Applied Kinesiology. It is a simple, gentle, yet powerful technique that children and their families can use to manage their emotions, fears, traumas and even physical pain. Gentle tapping with the fingertips is used on specific points of the face and body while focusing on a specific problem, such as fear, and stating phrases about that fear. This removes the energetic and emotional imbalance in the body that creates the fear.

How can this be? Well, the body's operating system is electrical and chemical. Thus, Tapping stimulates this electrical system positively, which in turn stimulates the body's natural chemical system. Instead of producing stress hormones and chemicals that weaken the immune system, the body thereby produces relaxing and healing hormones and chemicals that *strengthen* the immune system and improve health.

But first, a little background on the sympathetic and parasympathetic nervous systems. The sympathetic nervous system of the brain releases stress hormones, such as cortisol and adrenaline, in response to real danger, as well as to our negative and fearful emotions. They prepare the body for fight or flight by increasing heart rate, preparing muscles for physical activity and more. If the body is perpetually stressed out or on alert, one becomes more susceptible to illness, as this chronic stress reduces the overall strength of the immune system.

The parasympathetic nervous system of the brain, on the other hand, prepares the body for relaxation, cell regeneration and digestion, which strengthens the immune system. Scientific studies have indicated that EFT is helpful in boosting one's emotional and physical state of being by reducing the amount of cortisol released in the body (see References), thus aiding the parasympathetic nervous system.

PHYSICAL RECOVERY IS ENHANCED WITH A POSITIVE ATTITUDE

When dealing with a serious illness, it is important to have a strong immune system in order to aid recovery. It is well-known that a positive, cheerful attitude improves the immune system. Reducing feelings of fear, anxiety, anger and upset play an important part in helping the body to recover from a serious illness.

As mentioned above, it has been scientifically demonstrated (see References) that EFT or Tapping can calm the sympathetic nervous system, thus reducing stress hormones such as cortisol. In doing so, it allows the parasympathetic nervous system to actively help in the regeneration process, calming the mind and body and boosting the immune system. The body's natural default pathway is to heal. With EFT, it is possible to support that natural process as well as to feel good emotionally.

REAL-LIFE EXAMPLES

The stories in this book are based on children I have worked with in a hospital setting. These children were dealing with incredibly challenging real-life situations, ranging from fever to pain to the possibility of death. They used EFT or Tapping to relax, reduce pain and feel better emotionally.

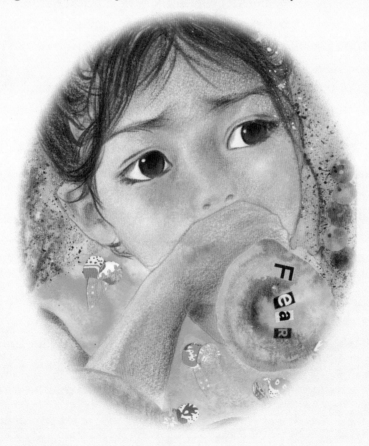

EFT IN A HOSPITAL — IMPROVING THE QUALITY OF LIFE OF CHILDREN WITH CANCER

How does one deal with the emotions that occur when one's child is diagnosed with a serious illness such as cancer? Anyone dealing with this situation knows that there are many moments of fear, anxiety, stress, pain, anger, frustration and more. Knowing how to manage these emotions allows people to improve their quality of life throughout the process of their journey with the illness.

There are many stress factors for children and their family members in any hospital setting. As well as the physical pain and worry, they are often far from home and their normal support network, which can make the experience seem even more scary and alienating. However, when children and their parents have a tool, such as EFT, that they can use to help them manage their emotions and to allow them to choose to feel calm, strong and powerful, then they are training their mind and body to feel better too.

WHY IS IT IMPORTANT TO MANAGE DIFFICULT EMOTIONS THAT ARISE FROM ILLNESS?

As mentioned above, improving mood also improves the immune system. If a child is sad and depressed, their immune system is weakened. The opposite is also true: if a child feels happy and cheerful, their immune system is strengthened.

By using EFT, children release the fears, anxieties and much of the pain associated with cancer. It helps them prepare for the treatments they'll receive and allows them to choose to be relaxed, so that these procedures are easier and more comfortable for them. EFT is completely complementary to all medical treatments given, meaning there are no negative side effects or interactions from using EFT.

BENEFITS OF TAPPING WITH CHILDREN

- ♥ Reduces stress and fear
- ♥ Reduces pain and nausea
- ♥ Eases the insertion of an IV
- ♥ Improves mood

♥ Gives the child a sense of empowerment
♥ Helps the child to visualize their healing process
♥ Provides them with a tool to manage their emotions
♥ Is fun to do and feels good

BENEFITS OF TAPPING WITH FAMILY MEMBERS

♥ Reduces stress, anxiety and worry
♥ Gives parents a useful tool to manage and improve their feelings while supporting their child through a serious illness
♥ Empowers parents to help themselves and help their child feel calm
♥ Allows parents to be more present for their children

A TOOL YOUR CHILD CAN USE TO RELEASE FEAR AND UPSET

Imagine a child who is fearful and anxious, calming down and beginning to play. That is exactly what happens when these children use Tapping.

One doesn't have to suffer to heal. The healing process can be filled with peace, joy, love and laughter. Tapping is one technique that helps make that possible.

WHAT TO EXPECT — INTRODUCING EFT TO CHILDREN, AND SUBSEQUENT BENEFITS

This book provides stories and Tapping sequences specifically related to various challenges that young children must deal with when facing cancer. Everything from fear to sadness, to pain and low functioning immune system, is addressed in the ten stories that follow. You will find that you can simply read and tap along with the stories together with your child. You are invited to answer the questions provided and follow the suggestions for how to make these stories fit more closely with your child's needs.

I generally introduce younger children to EFT by asking them if they are aware that they have 'Magic Fingers.' Most of them open their eyes wide and shake their heads no. I ask them if they'd like to learn how to use their Magic Fingers and they enthusiastically nod yes. From there, I show them how to tap by Tapping on myself or on them, with fun phrases and topics that raise their self-esteem. For example, "I'm a great kid," "I'm a wonderful boy/girl," or "I'm amazing."

With older children, I explain how they can be in control of their emotions, making them feel more powerful. I use their own words and images to help them connect with their emotions in order to release any trauma and become calm. If necessary, I can explain to them in simple scientific terms, how EFT works.

I find most children are open to doing something fun like Tapping, especially if they feel better while or after doing so.

Allowing children to use their imagination is essential. They can use it to help them have an image of being pain-free, of healing their bodies, of feeling happier, or playful. Allow your child to enjoy Tapping — play with it, change it around and make the statements his or her own. Have fun with Tapping and let it take you to amazing places within yourself, bringing back the joy and laughter.

Laughing in itself has a great number of health benefits and is important in the recovery process. It helps the body boost the immune system by decreasing stress hormones and increasing immune cells and antibodies. It relaxes the body and relieves physical tension, as well as increasing blood flow. Laughing also causes the body to release endorphins, temporarily relieving pain and promoting a sense of wellbeing.

Since I started using EFT or Tapping at the hospital, the sound of laughter is often heard in the children's cancer ward.

THINGS TO BE AWARE OF WHEN USING EFT WITH CHILDREN

Tapping is extremely flexible. I use many images along with the technique itself, because children are very visual. Many of them don't know what they are feeling but they can identify a color or shape that represents it. Simply ask them, "What color or shape is the pain?" "What color or shape is the thing, emotion or person that bothers you?" Then they can tap on changing that color or shape from something ugly or unpleasant into something beautiful that makes them feel better.

Be aware that each child is unique and therefore the way in which they use EFT will also be unique to them. There are some children who, from the moment you mention Magic Fingers, are off and tapping. They'll continue to tap with you or on their own. They truly have fun with it. Other children are more timid and it takes time for them to trust you and connect with this technique, but as they begin to feel safe with it and feel better on all levels, they too will continue. Some children are resistant to Tapping because they think it looks 'weird,' but in private they tap because it helps them feel better.

Tapping for a child with cancer requires persistence, not only for the child but also for the parents. Do the Tapping on yourself daily. It is important for the parents to be calm in order to be able to better support their child. If you are a parent, remind your child to tap. Or better yet, let your child observe you using the technique. They are more likely to use it too if they see you use it. Tap with your child, as he or she will appreciate not only feeling better because of the technique, but also the connection with you, their parent.

Recognize that sometimes your child may not want to participate. As with all of us, sometimes we want to wallow in bad feelings, or it is just easier to stay angry or upset. You, as a parent, can gently show them how much better it feels to use Tapping and let go of those unwanted emotions.

In some instances, you can tap on yourself about how your child is still wonderful even if he or she doesn't want to tap. Many times they will begin to tap with you. Other times, you can play with them or just hold them and gently tap on them. On certain occasions, you won't want to tap with them at that moment but rather wait a little while before tapping. No matter how your child responds, be gentle, be patient, and use Tapping on yourself in those moments.

As you do, you will feel calmer instead of frustrated, and that alone will help your child. When a parent is calm, the child calms, and vice versa. When a parent models to their child that taking care of one's emotions is important, the child will learn an important lesson — that one can choose to use tools such as Tapping in order to release unwanted emotions and feel calm, at peace, happy and filled with love.

ADAPTING THE TAPPING SCRIPTS IN THE STORIES TO BE AGE-SPECIFIC

Since the stories in this book are based on real-life Tapping experiences, the script in each story is specific to the age of the child with whom the Tapping was done. If you are using these scripts with a child who is younger or older, then make sure you adapt the wording so that it is age-appropriate for your child.

For example:

♥ 1-4 years old: I'm a good baby. I'm a good kid. I'm a good little girl or boy. I'm sweet and special. I'm precious.

♥ 5-10 years old: I'm a great child. I'm an amazing young girl or boy. I'm a super kid. I'm so special. I'm so loveable. I'm adorable.

♥ 10-12 years old: I'm a smart kid, an amazing kid, a wonderful girl or boy. I'm magnificent. I have my own special talents. I'm amazing and I'm smart.

♥ 13-18 years old: I'm special just because I'm me. I'm an intelligent teen. I'm a remarkable young man or woman. I'm doing my best and will continue to do even better. I'm determined to get better. I will do whatever is necessary to get better.

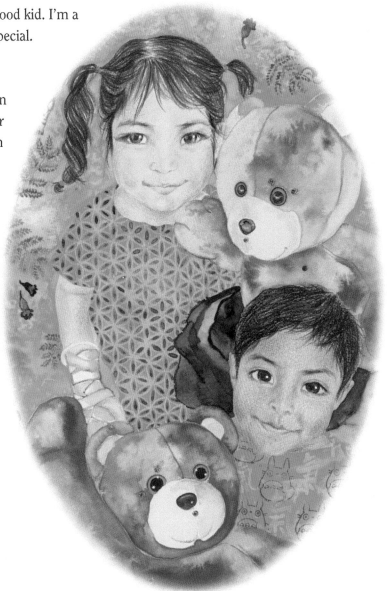

TAPPING POINTS

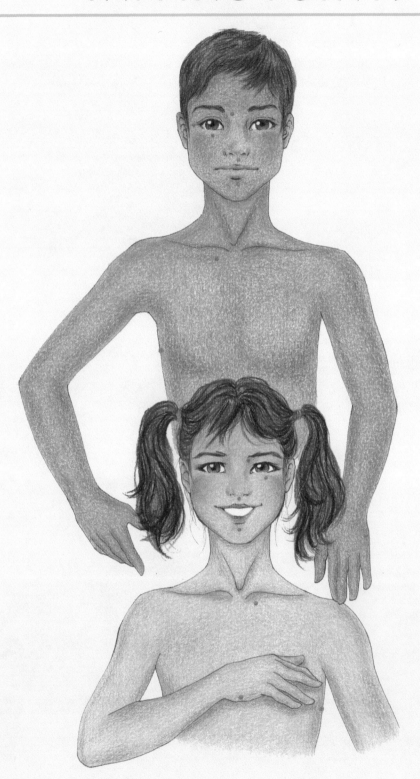

HOW TO TAP

*W*ith EFT or Tapping, one taps lightly with the tips of 2-3 fingers on either hand on particular points on the head, body and hands (on either side of the body), while at the same time saying words and phrases that describe the emotions or issue at hand. By doing so, our thoughts and emotions calm, allowing the mind and body to feel better.

Tap (a light, gentle tap-tap-tapping) on each of the following points while repeating the phrases in this book. You will soon see how easy it is and how good it feels.

- ♥ Karate Chop Point
- ♥ Eyebrow
- ♥ Side of the Eye
- ♥ Under the Eye
- ♥ Under the Nose
- ♥ Chin
- ♥ Collarbone
- ♥ Under the Arm
- ♥ Top of the Head

THE 0 TO 10 SCALE

Use a scale to determine the amount of pain, or emotion such as fear, that your child feels. This numerical scale goes from 0 to 10, where 0 means that he or she feels no pain or emotional charge, and 10 is the maximum amount of pain or emotion. Every number in between represents an intermediate intensity level of pain or emotion.

Ask your child how much pain they feel. The answer is subjective, but it can be used to aid Tapping, by helping the child recognize when a shift or reduction in intensity of pain or fear has occurred. This knowledge helps the child feel better.

If your child is too young to answer with a number to represent how strongly they feel an emotion, you can simply have them extend their arms to show how big or small the pain or emotion is. Hands together represent a 0 and arms extended as far apart as possible represent a 10. Anything in between represents intermediate values.

Most of the time, when tapping, the emotional intensity drops and continues to drop until zero is reached. Occasionally, the emotion intensifies before it goes down, which indicates that the emotion is shifting. If the

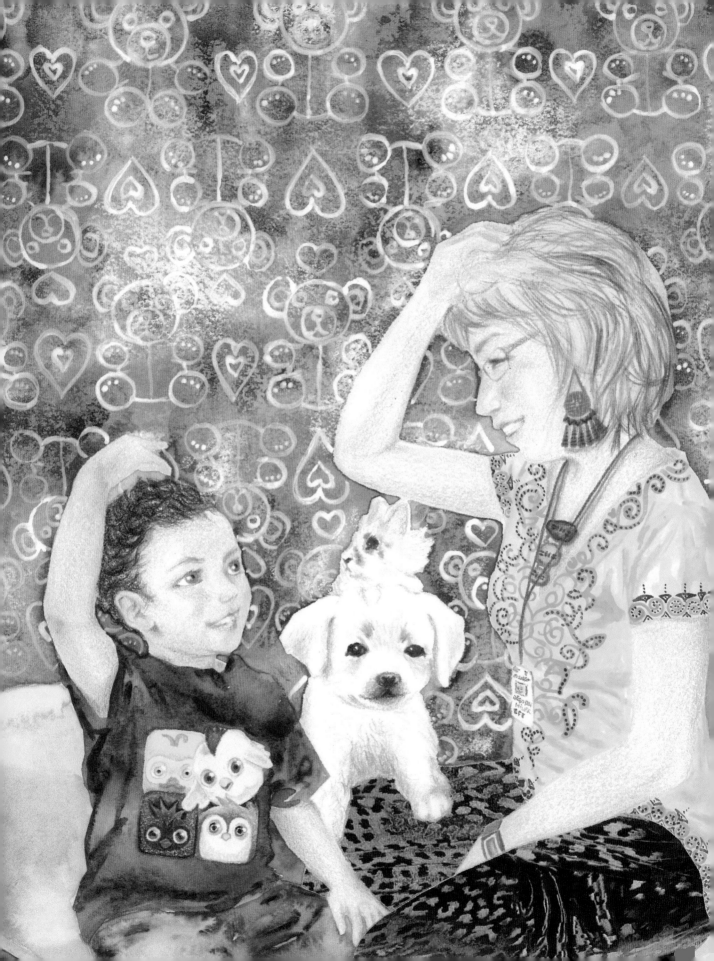

number representing an emotion doesn't change then it implies that the words being used aren't connecting with the experienced emotion, or a different issue is underlying the problem. Change the wording or topic.

BASIC TAPPING STEPS

♥ Identify the issue at hand (emotion, problem or what's bothering you or your child).

♥ Rate how strong that issue is on an intensity scale of 0-10. (Using a number scale or outstretched hands.)

♥ Gently tap each of the EFT tapping points in sequence while stating phrases about the issue out loud. Tap five to seven times on each point using the tips of 2-3 fingers.

♥ Take a deep breath.

♥ Again, rate the intensity of the issue on the intensity scale of 0-10.

♥ Repeat until the intensity drops to zero, or move on to another issue.

TWO EXAMPLES OF HOW I USE EFT WITH CHILDREN

Negative to Positive Phrasing: In the first rounds, tap while saying phrases that describe the issue (negative emotions or problem such as fear or pain). Once the initial emotional intensity drops to a 2-3 on the intensity scale, then you can begin to use more positive words and phrases until the intensity drops to zero.

Images and Colors: Since most children are visual and don't have the skill to describe their emotions, I use a lot of images and colors to represent their emotions or issues. For example, 'fear' could be represented by the color black or a bad dog. Then tap along with the child using that color or image, eventually changing it from negative to positive.

TAPPING TOGETHER

I recommend that you, the parent, tap along with your child, saying the phrases for the child to repeat after you. This is easier for the child. An added bonus is that as you tap along with your child, you receive the relaxation effects for yourself as well. This is called 'borrowing benefits.'

Although EFT is a simple to use technique that even children can master, there is an art to it – the wording. This is an art that develops with practice and is enhanced by focusing on the emotions. Relax and tap. You can't really do it incorrectly, but with practice you will learn how to do it better and better.

HOW A PARENT CAN TAP — A SAMPLE TAPPING

One very important, yet frequently overlooked need, when taking care of a child with cancer, is for the parents to take care of themselves. It is so easy to focus first and foremost on the child. In my work at the hospital, I have seen over and over again parents who are feeling so stressed, anxious, worried and fearful that they are not able to be as helpful to their child as they could be. They are emotionally and physically exhausted, they get sick with colds more frequently, and they aren't emotionally present for their child. Obviously, this is contrary to what a parent desires, yet it's easy to forget that one must take care of oneself in order to take care of somebody else.

In order for me to teach you, the parent, how to teach your child to tap, I've decided to give you an experience of how EFT can help you relax and be in the best shape in order to care for your child. Let's tap now to reduce your worries and stress, in order for you to be completely present with your child.

REDUCING STRESS AND WORRY FOR PARENTS

Use the tips of 2-3 fingers to gently tap on each point shown in the diagram and repeat the phrases below.

ROUND 1

Tap on the Karate Chop Point and say (out loud if possible, otherwise mentally):
Even though I feel a lot of stress, I'm a good person.
Even though I feel so stressed going to the hospital all the time, I'm a great person.
Even though I have all of this stress dealing with this illness, I accept myself.

Eyebrow: All of this stress.
Side of the Eye: I have so much stress.
Under the Eye: I can't handle all of this stress.
Under the Nose: I'm exhausted from all the stress.
Chin: My body is filled with stress.
Collarbone: I don't know how to manage this stress.
Under the Arm: It feels like it is taking over.
Top of the Head: All the stress I feel right now.

ROUND 2

Eyebrow: I have so much stress.
Side of the Eye: This illness has changed my life completely.
Under the Eye: Our lives are not the same at all.
Under the Nose: Everything is different.

Chin: Our life goals have changed.

Collarbone: Our work has changed.

Under the Arm: Our daily routine has changed.

Top of the Head: I don't recognize anything anymore.

ROUND 3

Eyebrow: It is all so strange.

Side of the Eye: I still can't accept it sometimes.

Under the Eye: I just want my child to get better.

Under the Nose: I worry. I worry a lot, about everything from a simple sniffle, to shots, and trips to the hospital.

Chin: I worry about my child's defenses — are they strong enough?

Collarbone: I worry about the money and time it costs us.

Under the Arm: It's normal for a parent to worry, isn't it?

Top of the Head: The problem is that worry just lowers my defenses and doesn't really solve anything.

ROUND 4

Eyebrow: Worrying too much will just stress me out and lower my defenses.

Side of the Eye: All this stress and worry won't help my child.

Under the Eye: I want to help my child by not being all stressed out.

Under the Nose: I want to find a way to get rid of my worry and stress.

Chin: Worry lowers my defenses and I want to be strong for my child.

Collarbone: Worry and stress make me uncertain and indecisive when I want to be clear and strong.

Under the Arm: Worry is just my thoughts going round and round and round.

Top of the Head: That makes me foggy-headed instead of clear-minded and focused.

ROUND 5

Eyebrow: I would like to do things that get rid of this worry.

Side of the Eye: I'm not exactly sure how it works, but Tapping calms my mind and body.

Under the Eye: That's a good start, to release my stress and worry.

Under the Nose: I can teach my child how to relax too. That's a double bonus.

Chin: Today, I choose to do what is best for my child and for me.

Collarbone: I choose to manage my emotions so that I can be the best support possible for my child.

Under the Arm: As I tap today, I choose to let go of some worry and stress.

Top of the Head: I would like to calm my mind, even if I don't really know how to do so.

ROUND 6

Eyebrow: I choose to lower the number of thoughts raging through my mind.

Side of the Eye: I imagine that I have a control knob that lowers their volume.

Under the Eye: I reduce the speed and number of thoughts racing through my mind.

Under the Nose: I use an imaginary dial where I turn down the volume and number of thoughts in my mind.

Chin: All those thoughts and feelings about my child that make me worried and stressed.

Collarbone: It doesn't help me at all to have all those thoughts racing through my mind. It is better to reduce them so I can think clearly.

Under the Arm: I choose to tone them down so that I can be present for my child.

Top of the Head: I choose to let go of some of the stress stored in my body too.

ROUND 7

Eyebrow: One of the best things I can do for my child is to take care of myself.

Side of the Eye: If I'm in good shape – physically and emotionally – then I will be more loving and present for my child.

Under the Eye: I choose to breathe deeply. I choose to worry less and have more faith.

Under the Nose: I choose to be positive and look at the bright side of things.

Chin: I choose to eat well so I stay healthy. I choose to help my child eat well too.

Collarbone: I choose to laugh and smile so that my child will feel happier.

Under the Arm: Being happy is such a great help to our defenses. I choose to bring in joy even now.

Top of the Head: These are things I can do to be healthy and supportive of my child. I choose to do so, because it is that important to me.

Take a deep breath. And another. Next, take a drink of water. It's important to breathe fully and stay hydrated when doing EFT. Always have a glass of water on hand and take a sip after each round if possible. At the end, take a few deep breaths.

How do you feel now, after this short example of Tapping to release stress and worry? Much calmer, I hope.

EFT helps one quickly take the edge off by lowering the stress hormone levels in the body. It also helps one find and release emotions that are hidden, or are consciously being held in. In this case, Tapping may bring up some emotion initially but then it will drop off. Don't worry if this happens — all you need to do is keep tapping and you will calm down within a few seconds or minutes, leaving you feeling much better. Sometimes you need to do several rounds of Tapping. It's totally normal.

Tap a few minutes each day and you'll find that you will be able to peacefully share your feeling of love and calm with your child.

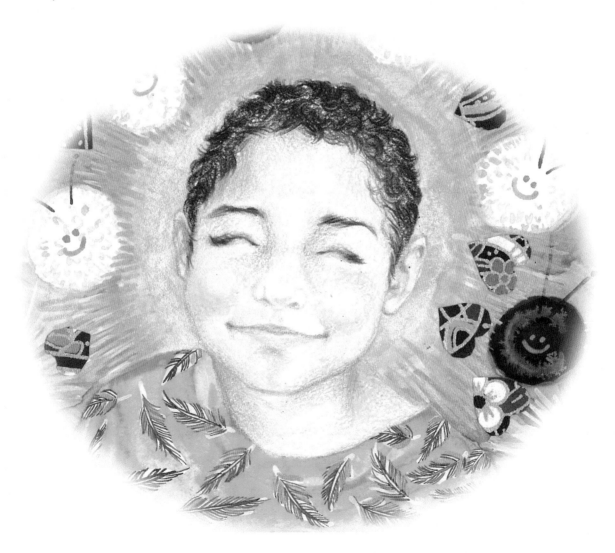

TAPPYBEAR — A TAPPING PARTNER

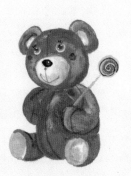

TappyBear is a stuffed teddy bear that was created specifically to use with EFT or Tapping. He has buttons on his body in the same spots as the Tapping points on a person. The reason I enjoy using TappyBear so much is that he is soft and cuddly and he looks at you as you are Tapping. He gives comfort to the children by his presence and by the fact that he reminds them to tap in order to feel better. These things combine to make him a valuable asset for improving the quality of life for children with serious illness.

JACARANDA TREE

It's a wonderful idea to have a symbol that represents your inner strength and power. For the children at the hospital and I, this symbol is the Jacaranda tree, a large tree with marvelous lavender-colored flowers. "Why?" you may ask. Well, it's because there is a Jacaranda tree outside the hospital that stands tall and strong to remind the children every day of this strength and power.

It has beautiful flowers, so it reminds them of the beauty of life and living. The lavender color of the blossoms is also a powerful healing color. The Jacaranda tree is peacefully growing with inner strength, while providing shade from the hot sun, and sharing its glorious color no matter what is going on around it.

The symbol of the Jacaranda tree is a reminder:

- to plant your roots; hold positive thoughts and feelings to maintain strength and the belief you will get better
- to have a trunk; your body supports you and keeps you upright
- to have branches; your arms and legs, as well as a positive attitude, let you expand and stretch yourself while growing healthier
- to have leaves; a healthy digestive system, absorbs the energy and power from the sun and food to strengthen your body. That requires eating healthy food like fresh green vegetables and fruit.

A picture of the Jacaranda tree will be found within this book to remind you to be strong, steady and powerful, like a beautiful tree. It will remind you that you are supported and cared for.

Each day remember the Jacaranda tree. Feel as if you are under its branches or leaning on its strong and supporting trunk. Even if you are in the hospital, you can imagine yourself outside sitting under the Jacaranda tree, where you are safe and peaceful and sheltered.

Come under the Jacaranda tree with TappyBear and I, and enjoy the journey of learning how to improve your life with Tapping.

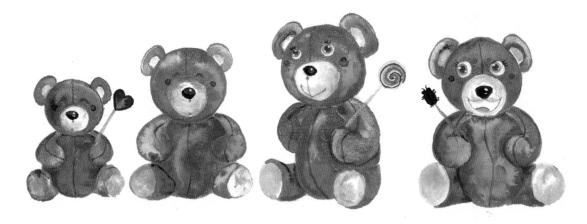

INDIVIDUAL STORIES

Based on a Child's
Experience

(plus Tapping Scripts)

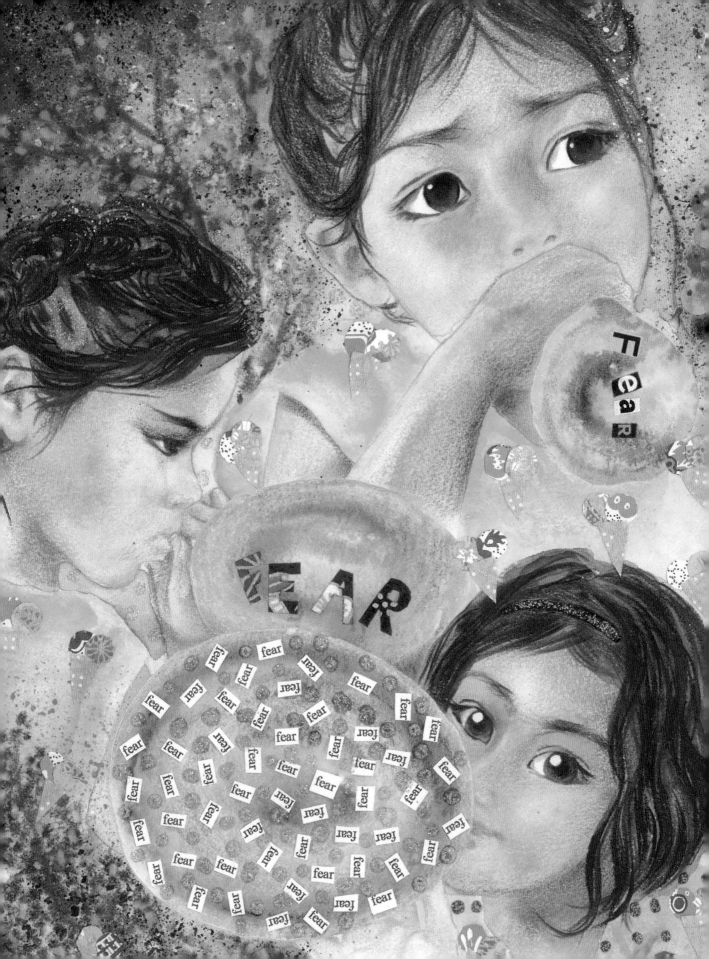

BALLOONS, BALLOONS, BALLOONS!

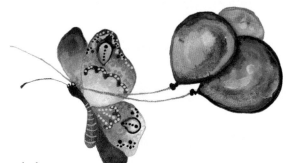

*B*alloons, balloons, balloons!!! Balloons of all colors help you get rid of your fears. Balloons come in all sizes and colors to help you face what's bothering you.

Gilda was always afraid. She was afraid of everything at the hospital. She was afraid before anything had even happened. She would imagine what *might* happen and feel afraid. Most of the time, she was afraid even when she didn't need to be. It wasn't any fun.

Gilda didn't want to be afraid anymore so we used Tapping with the image of balloons to help her feel better. Tap with us to get rid of your fears too.

Imagine a fear that you have. See it and feel it. Now imagine that you can put that fear inside an imaginary balloon. Imagine that balloon is in front of you. You can make the balloon any color, shape or size that you want.

What color is your balloon? Is it a plain color, or is it striped, or with stars or spots or something else on it? How big is your balloon? Is it small or is it as big as a house?

Now that you have that imaginary balloon with you, tap along and we'll put your fear inside the balloon. Remember — you are imagining these balloons. You don't need to have a real balloon in front of you.

ROUND 1

Tap on the Karate Chop point and say:

Even though I feel so afraid, I'm a great kid.

Even though I feel afraid of what is happening to me, I'm a wonderful kid.

Even though I'm afraid of all the scary things in my head, I want to feel better.

Eyebrow: I'm so scared. I don't know what to do.

Side of the Eye: I am so afraid. This fear is so BIG!

Under the Eye: What do I do with all of this fear?

Under the Nose: The fear is in my head.

Chin: The fear is in my mind and thoughts.

Collarbone: The fear is in my body.

Under the Arm: I am so afraid.

Top of the Head: This fear is so BIG!

ROUND 2

Eyebrow: I don't know how to feel better, but I want to feel better.

Side of the Eye: I have a great imagination, so I can think of a way to get rid of these fears.

Under the Eye: I know — I can put them in an imaginary balloon and send them away.

Under the Nose: I have a BIG BLUE balloon (or whatever color you want to imagine). I put my fear in a BLUE balloon.

Chin: I blow and blow and blow all of my fear into the big blue balloon.

Collarbone: The blue balloon gets bigger and bigger as my fear fills it up.

Under the Arm: When it is full of all of my fear, I tie it off.

Top of the Head: I let it go — why not? — and it floats up into the sky and disappears. Yeah!!

ROUND 3

Eyebrow: That feels so much better.

Side of the Eye: My mind is quieter but I still have a teensy, weensy bit of fear left.

Under the Eye: I want to get rid of it too, because I don't like fear.

Under the Nose: I get out an imaginary PINK balloon. A beautiful PINK balloon with swirls on it.

Chin: I blow and blow and blow all the rest of my fear into the balloon.

Collarbone: The balloon gets fatter and fatter as I put all the rest of my fear into it.

Under the Arm: I'm so glad I can put my fear in the balloon.

Top of the Head: I put every little tiny bit of my fear into the pink balloon and then I tie it off, and let it float away.

ROUND 4

Eyebrow: I feel so much better now. No more fear.

Side of the Eye: I have all the balloons I need to get rid of any fears I have.

Under the Eye: That makes me feel really safe.

Under the Nose: I have red balloons, white balloons, pink balloons, purple balloons, yellow balloons, green balloons, orange balloons, striped balloons, flowered balloons, balloons with stars and spots on them — any kind I want.

Chin: It is so easy to put all of my troubles into balloons and let them float up into the sky and disappear.

Collarbone: I'm so glad I have balloons to help me feel better.

Under the Arm: Now I feel light and free and happy!

Top of the Head: Balloons make me feel happy.

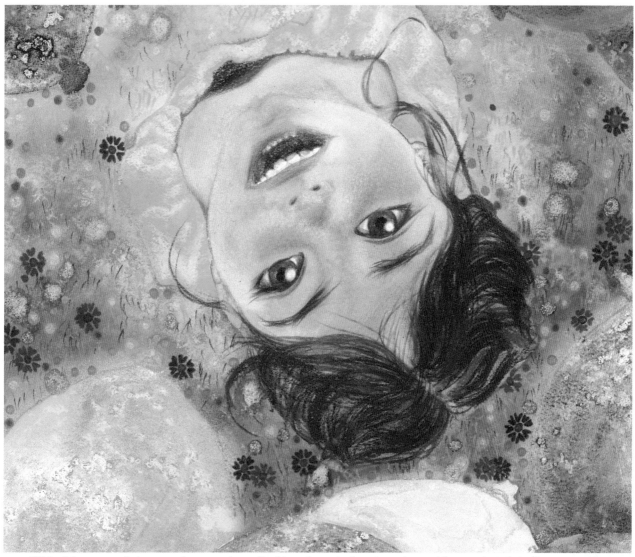

Gilda felt so much better after putting all of her fears in her imaginary blue and pink balloons and letting them disappear up into the sky. It only took two balloons to get rid of her fear. Now she knows that anytime she has a fear she can pick out another imaginary balloon and get rid of it. Sometimes it only takes one balloon, sometimes three. But no matter how many balloons it takes, she can get rid of her fear.

How about you? Do you feel better? Did your balloon help you get rid of a fear? Did you lose all your fears? If not, then get out another balloon and tap again until they are gone. If they are gone — YAY!!! You are amazing!

Remember any time you feel fear, you can put it in an imaginary balloon and send it away. You can put mad, sad and bad feelings in a balloon too and send them away. There are enough balloons to get rid of any unwanted feelings you may have.

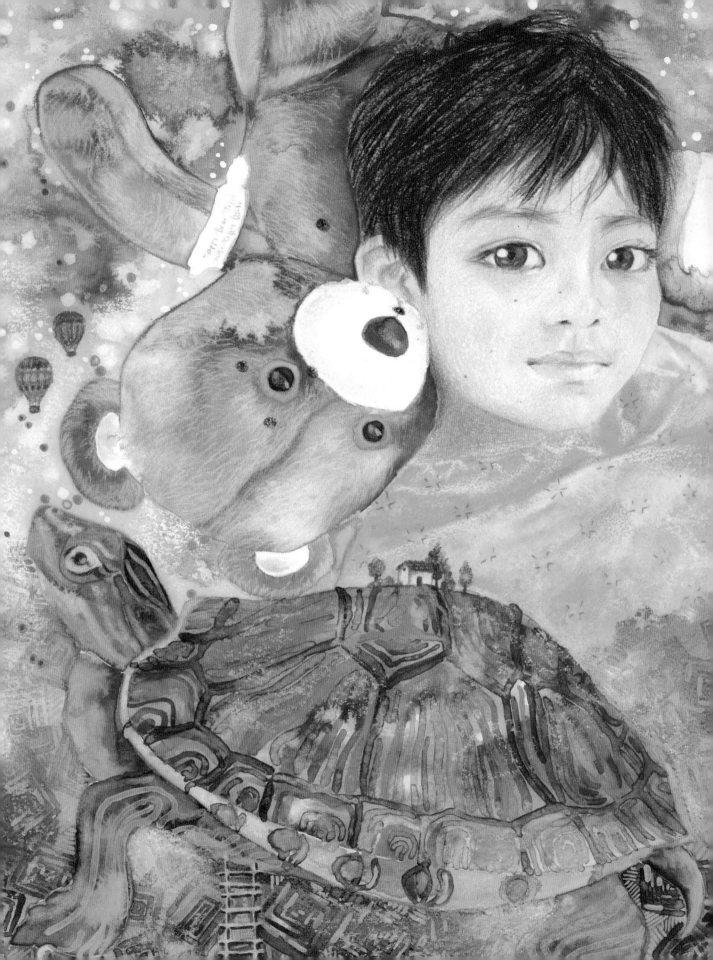

SLOW TURTLE AND FAST CHEETAH

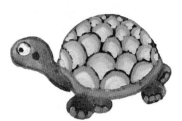

*Y*ou are still strong, even when you are healing from an illness. It is important to remember this. Your body has an immune system with many defenses. They are there to defend you, to take care of you and to help you get better when you feel sick. When your defenses are weak they can't do their job properly. They can't get rid of the bad bugs that make you have a cold. They can't make sure you pop back up after a chemotherapy treatment. They can't make you strong and full of energy. They can't do a very good job of making you healthy and keeping you that way.

What do you do when your defenses are down, and acting weak and wimpy? When your defenses are weak or can't do their job, we can give them a little help. Want to help your defenses be STRONG? Then come on this journey with Javier and I.

Javier's story is a perfect example of how to improve your defenses. This is his story. Javier was doing very well. He was getting better and better. He was very happy about that. He'd come into the hospital with a smile and make everyone laugh with his antics.

Then he had an appendicitis attack and had to have his appendix out. The surgery was really hard on his body. His defenses got weaker and weaker. His defenses just didn't snap out of it.

In fact, his chances of surviving dropped from 80/20 to 50/50. That was really depressing for Javier. He felt extremely sad and lost much of his hope. Instead of making people smile when he came to the hospital, he was all hunched over and sad. His big brown eyes looked down and almost dripped with sadness.

Because Javier's immune system was low and slow to react, he wasn't allowed to receive his cancer treatments so he could continue getting better. He felt worried about it. You could see in his big brown eyes that he knew this was not a good thing.

Here's what Javier did.

Javier and I tapped to give his defense system a boost to get it going again.

Tap along with the script below to help your defenses remember how strong they are.

ROUND 1

Tap on the Karate Chop point and say:

Even though I have low defenses and I can't have my treatments because of it, I'm a great kid.

Even though I feel sad because my defenses are low, and that isn't good, I'm still a wonderful kid.

Even though my immune system is weak and that is bad if you want to get better, I'm a great, great kid.

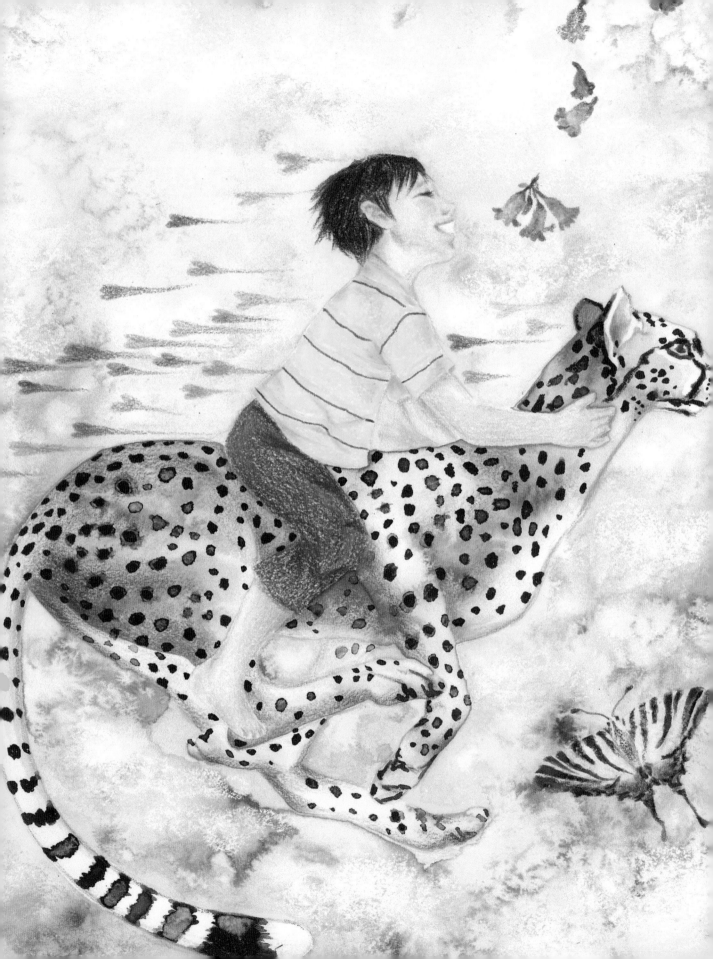

Eyebrow: I feel sad because my defenses are down.

Side of the Eye: I don't want them to be weak and slow.

Under the Eye: It makes me so, so sad that they are weak. It scares me.

Under the Nose: I know it is not good to have weak defenses.

Chin: I don't want my defenses to be slow like a turtle.

Collarbone: Being slow like a turtle won't help me get better.

Under the Arm: Turtles are great and they have a strong shell, but they are just too slow and I want to get better fast!

Top of the Head: I want my defenses to be as fast as a cheetah, because the cheetah is the fastest animal on the earth.

ROUND 2

Eyebrow: I want defenses that are fast and strong like a cheetah.

Side of the Eye: That will get my defenses moving just the way a cheetah can go from sitting to practically flying over the land.

Under the Eye: I ask that my defenses get up and get moving fast because they are aware of their surroundings and what is needed — just like a cheetah.

Under the Nose: My defenses like being strong, fast, and adjust to whatever they need to do in a flash.

Chin: I like having strong and fast defenses like a cheetah.

Collarbone: I like feeling fast and full of energy and speed like a cheetah.

Under the Arm: My defenses respond and get moving fast — right now.

Top of the Head: That makes me strong and powerful.

ROUND 3

Eyebrow: Being strong and powerful lets my defenses do their job — DEFEND ME!

Side of the Eye: I like that my defenses take care of me.

Under the Eye: They get rid of the bad stuff and make me feel better.

Under the Nose: I am glad that I have strong defenses.

Chin: I let the defenses that are slow like a turtle get fast like a cheetah.

Collarbone: Instead of slow defenses like a turtle, I have fast defenses like a cheetah.

Under the Arm: My defenses get fast and strong like a cheetah.

Top of the Head: My defenses are fast and strong like a cheetah, making me strong. Whoo hoo!!

ROUND 4

Eyebrow: Having strong and speedy defenses like a cheetah keeps me strong.

Side of the Eye: I love being strong because it helps me be healthy.

Under the Eye: My cheetah defenses keep me strong.

Under the Nose: Having strong defenses makes me healthier and healthier.

Chin: I want to be healthy. I like being healthy.

Collarbone: I love having my cheetah defenses making sure I'm strong.

Under the Arm: I love being strong and healthy like a cheetah.

Top of the Head: My body and I are strong and healthy like a cheetah.

Javier and I tapped on a Thursday afternoon and by Monday his defenses were strong and fast. You can do the same. Tap strong and healthy defenses into your body.

NOTE: Remember that these are the words that Javier and I used to help his defenses get moving. You can follow along and use these words exactly as they are, or you can use others words for 'defenses.' You can always adapt a Tapping script to fit your own personal situation in a way that rings true for you.

What word means 'defenses.' for you? What images make you feel STRONG — a superhero? A superboy or supergirl? A different animal?

Perhaps you'd like to imagine your defenses are like a castle: a great big complex castle with a moat around it and hundreds of warriors waiting to defend it. Some of these warriors are archers standing behind the battlements, ready to shoot down their arrows on any intruders. Some are foot soldiers, with swords, shields, helmets and armor. There are different kinds of soldiers that wear different uniforms and some of them even have X-ray glasses!

In the forest around the castle there are many wild animals that are all working with the warriors to help protect the castle in their own way. There is the Turtle, which is slow but has a strong, impenetrable shell. There is the Mama Bear, who stands tall, roars and chases intruders away. There are Wolves and Wild Cats that growl, bite and swat with their claws. And then there is the Cheetah, which runs as fast as the wind and nothing can escape it.

Be creative and use words and images that make *you* feel better. There is no limit – your imagination is free to fly, create and find images that are just right *for you*!

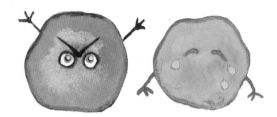

SAD CELLS GET HAPPY

Your body is unique and special. It is made up of many cells.

You may wonder, "What is a cell?" Cells are the smallest living part in your body. Each cell is like a room in your house. All the other cells are like the other rooms in your house. All of them together make up your house or your body.

Each cell is unique and special but is part of the house. Inside each room or cell is all the necessary stuff that helps your body eat, breathe, move, sleep, smile, cry, be strong and healthy, and everything else. Cells are the reason you are alive.

Cells talk to each other. They tell each other what's going on inside and around them. That means your cells know when you feel happy because they feel it. They know when you are sad too. Cells listen to how you feel and then tell each other what they need to make to be sad or happy, just like you.

You are the boss of your cells!

When you feel sad, your cells make chemicals that make your body feel sad too. The neat part is that when you are happy, your body makes chemicals that make your body feel happy too. Wow! That means you are so powerful — you can help your body feel better just because you choose to be happy!

For example, when you are sick, parts of your body are really sad because they don't feel good. All the other cells hear that. The good thing is you can help your body. When you decide to feel happy, the sad parts begin to feel happy too because your cells are listening to your happy thoughts and feelings. That helps your cells get better, and that helps your body get better too.

Let's help your cells get happy so that they can feel better and you can get better. Let's do Tapping with our magic fingers and magic wands to be happy.

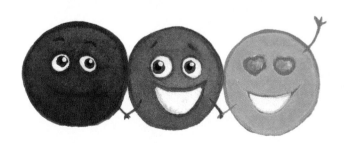

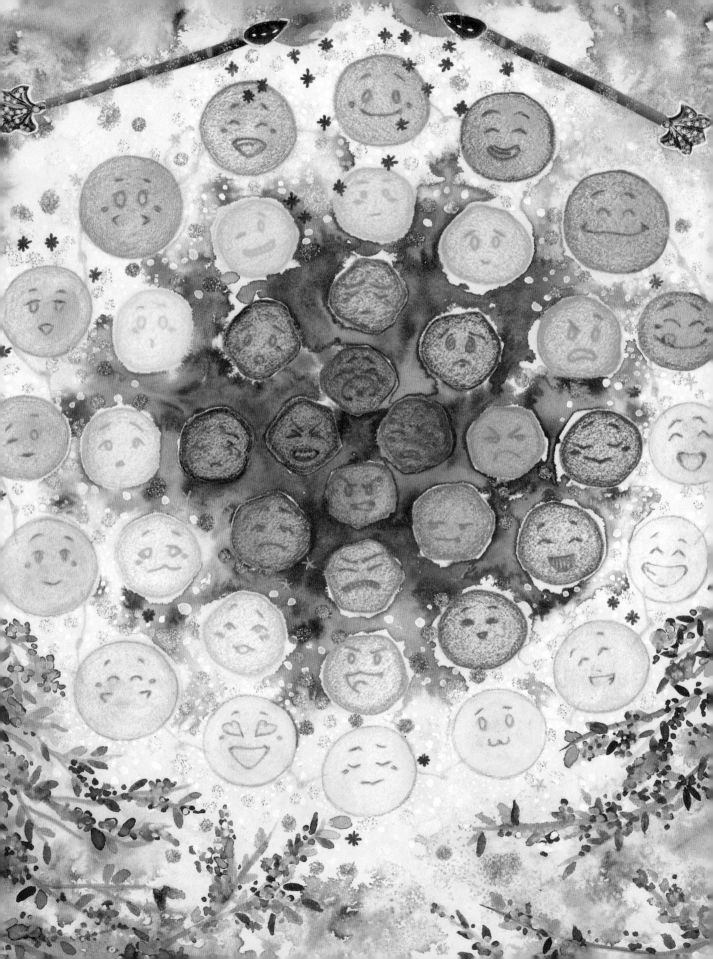

MAKING YOUR MAGIC WAND

You didn't know that you would be using a magic wand today, did you? Well, surprise! You can make your magic wand any way you want, because it's your special wand.

- ♥ Is it in your right hand or left hand?
- ♥ What color is it?
- ♥ How big is it?
- ♥ It is heavy or light?
- ♥ Does it glow in the dark?
- ♥ Is it a straight long stick or is there a star on the end of it? Or something else?
- ♥ Does it make sounds?
- ♥ Does it sparkle?

Now imagine you have a magic wand in your hand and let's make your cells happy.

ROUND 1

Tap on the Karate Chop point and say:
Even though I have sad parts, I'm a great kid.
Even though parts of my body are sick, and I don't know why, I'm still a great kid.
Even though parts of me are sad because they are sick, I'm a good kid.

Eyebrow: I am sad because I'm sick.
Side of the Eye: I don't want to be sick.
Under the Eye: Parts of my body are sad and sick.
Under the Nose: Part of my body is very, very sad that it got sick.
Chin: I don't want my body to be sick.
Collarbone: I want it to be better.
Under the Arm: I don't want sad cells.
Top of the Head: I want happy cells.

Imagine waving your magic wand as you tap!

ROUND 2

Eyebrow: I use my magic wand to remove the sadness from my cells.

Side of the Eye: My magic wand takes all the sadness out of me.

Under the Eye: It makes the sadness go PUFF! and disappear.

Under the Nose: PUFF! All gone! No more sadness!

Chin: I want my cells to be happy.

Collarbone: I'm going to use my magic wand and put happiness in my cells.

Under the Arm: Happiness is yellow for me. (Is it yellow for you? Or another color? You pick your color and use it — whichever color you want.)

Top of the Head: I put lots and lots and lots of happy yellow color in my cells.

ROUND 3

Eyebrow: Happy thoughts make my cells happy, too.

Side of the Eye: Glowing happy cells feel good and so do I.

Under the Eye: I love having happy, glowing cells, because they make me feel good.

Under the Nose: When I feel good, my cells feel good and I feel better.

Chin: My cells love feeling happy.

Collarbone: They fill up with happy yellow color and begin to glow.

Under the Arm: They glow with such happiness that I smile too.

Top of the Head: My cells are glowing with happy thoughts and feelings. I'm glowing too.

ROUND 4

Eyebrow: My cells and I are glowing with happy yellow thoughts.

Side of the Eye: All the cells in my body are glowing.

Under the Eye: This glow makes my body feel so good.

Under the Nose: This glow makes my sad cells feel good too.

Chin: Happy thoughts always make me feel better.

Collarbone: Happy thoughts make my cells happy too.

Under the Arm: That makes me glow and feel better.

Top of the Head: I love glowing every day.

Doesn't it feel good to glow and be happy? I'm sure your cells feel better too. Any time you feel sad, mad, hurt or upset, use your magic wand and put your favorite color in your thoughts and cells. Fill them up with that happy color. You'll be glowing and happy in no time. Whoo hoo!!!

WHAT TO DO WHEN YOU DON'T WANT TO GO TO THE HOSPITAL

Sometimes the hardest part of getting treatments at the hospital is going there. Who wants to go to a hospital?

It's not any fun at the hospital. There is pain there. There is fear there. I bet that sometimes you feel upset even before you go to the hospital. You might even fight with your parents about going to the hospital. That makes everyone sad.

A 10-year-old girl named Itzani felt like this. Normally at home she would be happy and playful but she became so sad every time she had to go to the hospital. This would happen days before she had to go. Instead of playing and doing things with her brother, she would mope around. She would get cranky and talk back to her mom. She would have the biggest frown ever. Her whole body looked sad too.

I asked Itzani:

"What if you could take your happy, fun, playful part of you to the hospital with you? Wouldn't that feel better? Let's tap to bring the fun part with you everywhere you go."

ROUND 1

Tap on the Karate Chop point and say:

Even though I don't want to go to the hospital, I'm a great kid.

Even though I don't want to go, I'm an amazing young person.

Even though I don't want to go, I'm so loveable.

Eyebrow: I don't want to go to the hospital.

Side of the Eye: It is horrible there.

Under the Eye: I feel upset, sad and mad there.

Under the Nose: I hate what happens to me there.

Chin: I get shots and meds that make me feel awful.

Collarbone: I don't want to go!!

Under the Arm: Don't make me go!!

Top of the Head: I want to stay home.

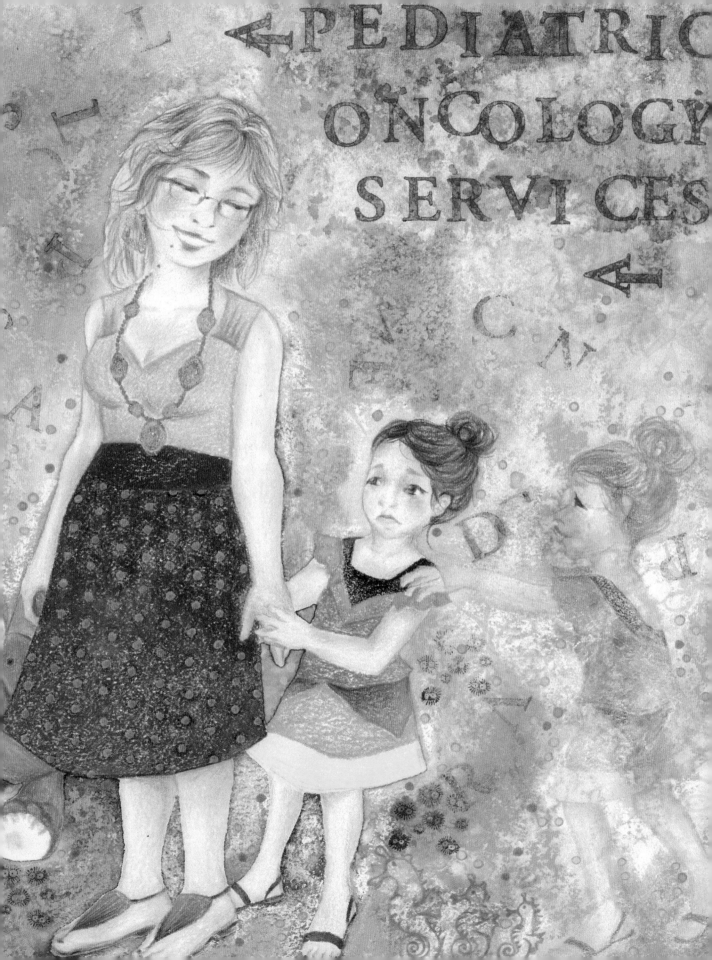

ROUND 2

Eyebrow: Of course I want to stay home.

Side of the Eye: I'm happier at home.

Under the Eye: It's more fun at home.

Under the Nose: Why would I want to go to the hospital?

Chin: I feel horrible there.

Collarbone: I'd rather play and have fun at home.

Under the Arm: I don't want to go someplace where I feel horrible.

Top of the Head: I'd rather not go to the hospital.

Take a deep breath. Just breathe — in… and out… How do you feel? Are you still mad that you have to go to the hospital? It's okay if you are. It's okay to not want to go. That's normal. Who wants to go to a hospital? Who wants to have chemo? It's more fun to play. It would be stranger if you jumped up and down and said you wanted to go to the hospital. But it would be better for you if you could go to the hospital calmly and without feeling upset.

So let's keep Tapping until you feel better.

ROUND 3

Eyebrow: I know I have to go.

Side of the Eye: I don't want to go.

Under the Eye: Just thinking about going to the hospital makes me sad.

Under the Nose: That doesn't help me get better.

Chin: I really want to get better.

Collarbone: I can tap to feel better about going to the hospital.

Under the Arm: I can tap about being happy wherever I am.

Top of the Head: Wow! That's pretty powerful. I'm in charge, not the hospital!

ROUND 4

Eyebrow: I can tap to feel better every day, everywhere.

Side of the Eye: I tap to feel happy because happiness is inside of me.

Under the Eye: Happiness lives inside of me. Fun lives inside of me.

Under the Nose: That means I can take it with me.

Chin: I can take happiness and fun everywhere I go.

Collarbone: Happiness and fun live right inside of me.

Under the Arm: I like being happy and having fun.

Top of the Head: I take my smile and laugh with me wherever I go.

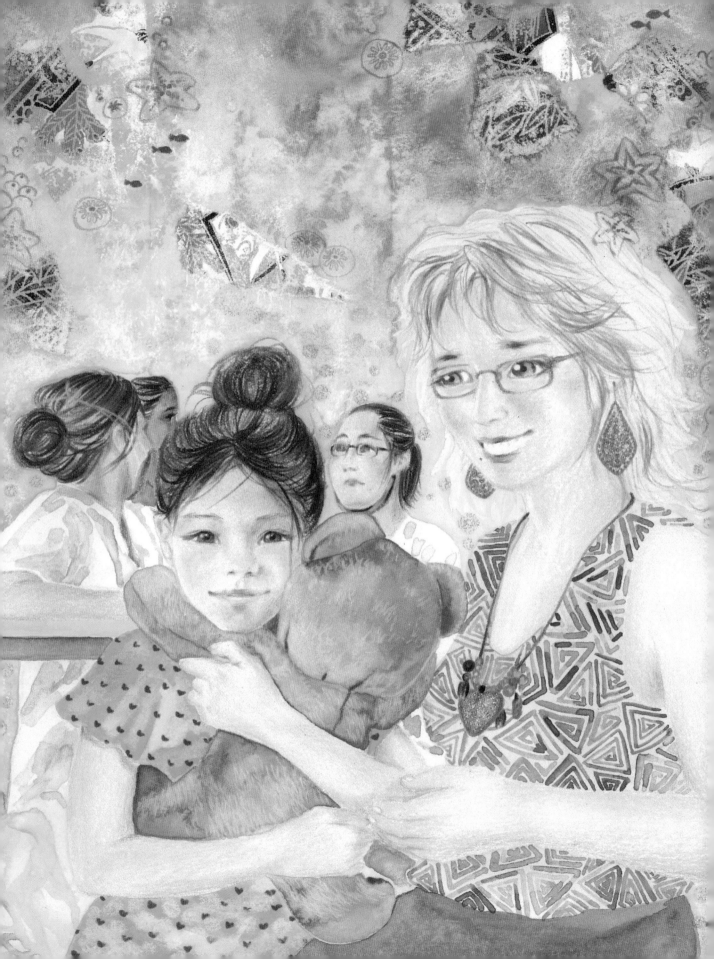

Imagine what that happy part inside of you looks like. Bring that image to mind and continue Tapping.

ROUND 5

Eyebrow: I can take my smile and laugh with me to school.
Side of the Eye: I can take my smile and laugh to the store or the park.
Under the Eye: I can even take my smile and laugh to the hospital.
Under the Nose: I would feel so much better if I had my smile with me.
Chin: Laughing and having fun even when I'm in the hospital would be fabulous.
Collarbone: I am really powerful because I can take the happy part of me with me.
Under the Arm: I choose to take my smile and laugh with me.
Top of the Head: That makes me feel better.

ROUND 6

Eyebrow: I share my smiles and laughs with everyone at the hospital.
Side of the Eye: That makes everyone at the hospital feel better too.
Under the Eye: It makes me happy.
Under the Nose: It makes the other kids happy.
Chin: It makes the other parents happy.
Collarbone: It makes the nurses and doctors happy too.
Under the Arm: I like that I can be happy anywhere I am.
Top of the Head: That makes me so powerful. I can be happy anywhere, every day! Whoo hoo!!!

Now that feels much better, doesn't it? Itzani found that she could bring the happy part of herself everywhere she went. Now she smiles wherever she is. She looks happier. She feels happier. And her body feels better, too.

She chooses to be happy at home, at school and even at the hospital. That makes her powerful, because she chooses to be happy wherever she goes. She brings joy with her and that helps everyone around her to be happier too.

Every morning, find the happy, fun part of yourself, and take it with you wherever you go. Pay attention to how you feel and what happens during the day when you bring this happy part along. Do you feel better? Do you enjoy the day? Do neat things happen when you bring your happy part with you instead of your grumpy, sad part? I bet they do.

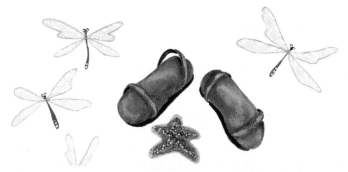

Enjoy your happy part. It's special and amazing, just like you.

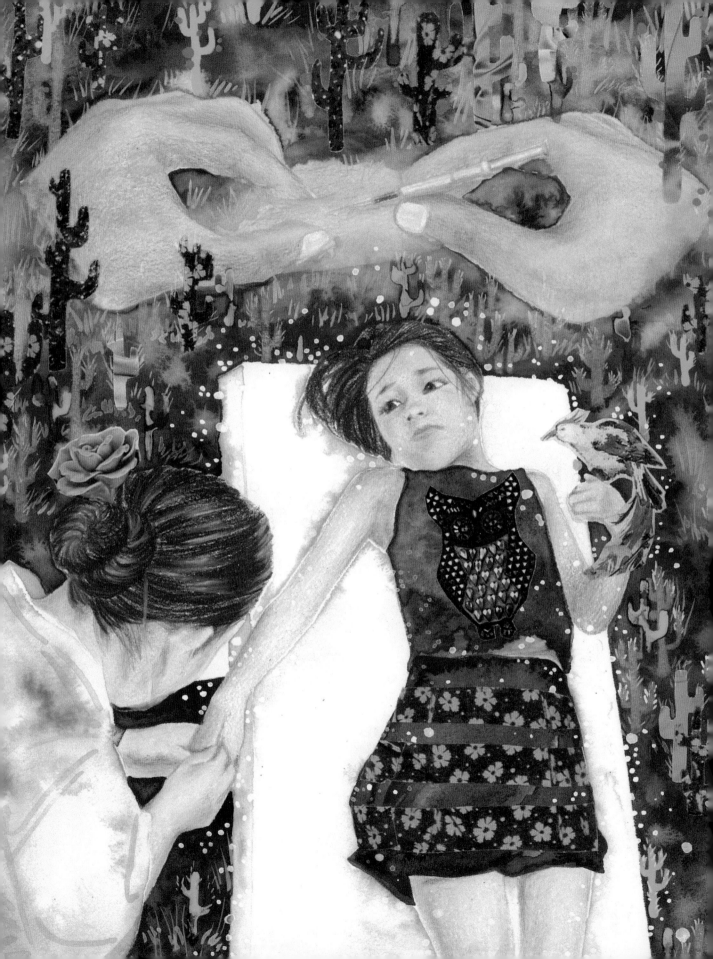

THE NEEDLE
AND THE BIG FAT VEIN

*M*arcelina hated needles. She used to fight with her family for days before she went to the hospital, because she didn't want to get poked with a needle.

Because she's a skinny girl, it was usually hard to find her veins. That meant she would get poked with the needle many times. She hated it. She would do just about anything to avoid it.

How about you? Are you afraid of getting a needle poke? It makes sense. No one likes it, but sometimes it is necessary. How would you like to feel when you go in for a shot? Wouldn't you like to be calm and relaxed instead of tense and afraid? Wouldn't it be great if you could get rid of some of that pain you feel when you get a shot — or better yet, have no pain at all when you get a shot? Do you think that's possible?

Try this and see what happens: think of something you hate, that makes you sad, or mad. Then look in the mirror and see what happens to the way your face looks. Does it look like a sad, mad or happy face?

How does your body feel — heavy or light? Do you feel worse or better? Do your muscles feel tight or relaxed?

Now think of something that makes you laugh and feel excited, or think of someone you love – maybe your mom or dad, your dog or cat, or having a birthday party or something you love to do. Look in the mirror again. Does your face look sad, mad or happy? Does your body feel heavy or light? Do you feel worse or better? Do your muscles feel tight or relaxed?

I bet you felt the difference! When you hated something, or were mad or sad, I bet you felt worse. But when you thought of laughing, being excited or thought about someone you love, you felt better. This means you are so powerful, you can make your body feel better!

Even when you get a shot, you can help your body relax. If your body is relaxed, then everything will go better.

One day I helped Marcelina tap so that it wouldn't be so painful while the nurse was putting in her IV. Marcelina's body was tense and her face was all scrunched up and tight because she was expecting pain.

I tapped with Marcelina about relaxing and having a big fat vein come to the surface so that it would be easy for the nurse to put in the IV needle. Marcelina relaxed, smiled and laughed as a big fat vein popped up. The nurse got the IV in on the first try, so Marcelina only had one poke that day. It was easy. That made her very happy.

Afterwards, Marcelina told me that she had been afraid when she got on the treatment table, like she always had been before, but when we tapped, she just forgot to be afraid. Her fear disappeared. Her body got calm. She felt as if her vein got bigger and that let the needle go in easier. She was very happy.

Marcelina's mother was very happy, too, to see her daughter so relaxed as the IV was put in — the last time she had one put in, it took three pokes before they found a good vein. She doesn't want to see her daughter hurting, so she was thankful that Tapping made it better for Marcelina. Tapping made her feel better, too, so everyone was happy.

Remember that Marcelina didn't believe it was possible to have a shot without pain until it happened to her. Now Marcelina wants to share with all kids who have to get shots that Tapping helps the mind and spirit relax and feel better. Then everything is easier. Tap along with us here and see what happens.

ROUND 1

Tap on the Karate Chop point and say:

I'm a great kid, even if I don't want to get a shot.

I'm a fabulous kid, even if I don't like needles.

I'm an awesome kid, even if I don't like shots.

Eyebrow: I don't want to go to the hospital.

Side of the Eye: I get poked every time I go there.

Under the Eye: I don't want to get up on that table.

Under the Nose: I know that something painful is coming.

Chin: I don't want to get a shot. It hurts a lot.

Collarbone: I won't let them do that to me.

Under the Arm: It scares me. I hate it.

Top of the Head: It hurts. I don't like it.

ROUND 2

Eyebrow: I'm scared for days before I have to get a shot.

Side of the Eye: I fight with my mom and dad because I don't want to go.

Under the Eye: I tell them I don't want to go, but they make me.

Under the Nose: They know it hurts me but they make me go.

Chin: That makes me mad too.

Collarbone: I don't want to go. I don't want to get a shot.

Under the Arm: They want me to get better, so they make me go.

Top of the Head: I want to get better too, so even though it hurts, I will go.

ROUND 3

Eyebrow: Getting poked with a needle hurts.

Side of the Eye: I don't want to get poked.

Under the Eye: But I do want to get better.

Under the Nose: I know the nurse doesn't want to hurt me.

Chin: The nurse wants me to get better too.

Collarbone: The nurse wants to get the vein on the first try too.

Under the Arm: The nurse only wants to poke me one time.

Top of the Head: We both want this to be easy.

ROUND 4

Eyebrow: I am a powerful kid, so I can make it better.

Side of the Eye: I am strong, so I choose to tap to feel better.

Under the Eye: Tapping makes me feel good.

Under the Nose: I relax when I tap.

Chin: I choose to relax so the needle doesn't hurt me.

Collarbone: I like when the needle doesn't hurt me.

Under the Arm: I know when I relax my body, it hardly hurts at all.

Top of the Head: I tap to relax so it doesn't hurt. That's cool!

ROUND 5

Eyebrow: If I relax my body it will be easier.

Side of the Eye: One way to relax is to breathe deeply.

Under the Eye: As I breathe deeply, my body relaxes.

Under the Nose: I take a really deep breath now. Ahhh!

Chin: Tapping makes my body relax even more!

Collarbone: When my body relaxes, my muscles relax.

Under the Arm: When my muscles relax, it is so easy for the needle to go in.

Top of the Head: It doesn't hurt then. I like that.

ROUND 6

Eyebrow: I know that if I feel scared, my body gets tense and tight.

Side of the Eye: I feel better knowing that I can breathe deeply and it helps me relax.

Under the Eye: I can choose to be calm. I remember to breathe because it relaxes me.

Under the Nose: I choose to relax and know that when I'm relaxed, it all goes better and faster.

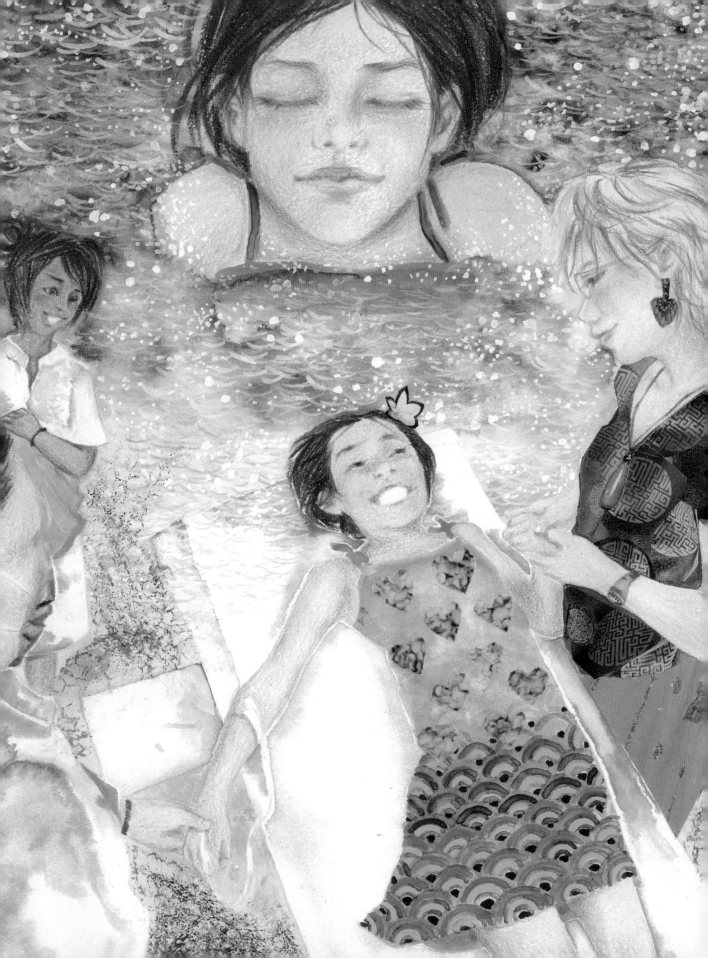

Chin: I want to remember to breathe deeply and tap, so that it doesn't hurt when I get poked with a needle.

Collarbone: I am so powerful. I can breathe, tap and talk to my body too.

Under the Arm: My body listens to me. It listens to what I tell it.

Top of the Head: I'm going to cooperate and talk to my veins.

ROUND 7

Eyebrow: I tell my veins that I don't want veins that are thin, and hide.

Side of the Eye: I want a vein that will be a volunteer, and pop up.

Under the Eye: I want a vein that says "Me! Me! I'll do it!"

Under the Nose: Then that vein comes to the surface.

Chin: That big fat vein is easy to see and easy to inject.

Collarbone: The nurse gets the big fat vein on the first try.

Under the Arm: The needle goes in so easily, I hardly feel it.

Top of the Head: I like that. It is easy. I want it to be like that every time.

ROUND 8

Eyebrow: I am calm, relaxed and have a big fat vein.

Side of the Eye: I know what to do to make it better. That makes me very powerful.

Under the Eye: I remember to breathe, tap and relax, and it's all over before I know it.

Under the Nose: I tell my body to send a big fat vein to the surface.

Chin: My vein listens. It pops right out. That big fat vein is easy to see.

Collarbone: It says, "Me! Me! I'm ready to help you." The nurse gets it on the first try.

Under the Arm: The needle goes in quickly and I'm done. Yeah!

Top of the Head: Wow! That was fast and easy. I say thanks to my vein for volunteering.

REMEMBER — you are powerful. You can help your body relax and feel better. You can choose to be calm. And now you know what to do, so every treatment you have will go better. Remember to breathe and tap every time you have to get poked with a needle, so that a big fat vein can pop up and it is easy and fast.

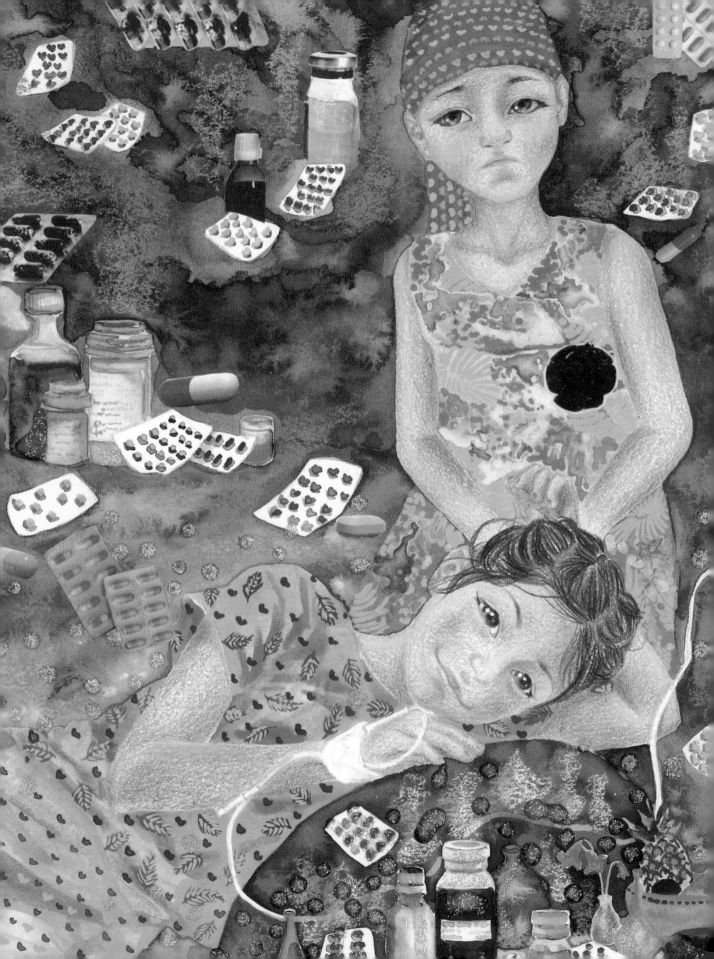

BAD MEDS HURT ME: USING EFT FOR STRONG NEGATIVE FEELINGS ABOUT DOCTORS, MEDS, OR DIFFICULT TREATMENTS

I bet that sometimes you get scared or angry when you have to go to the hospital for a treatment that hurts or makes you feel sick. Anyone can understand that. But even though it's understandable, it doesn't help you get better.

If you are afraid of your treatments, or hate them or the doctors, when you have to have the treatments anyway it REALLY makes you feel awful. Right?

Many times it's our thoughts that cause us to feel awful. If you have thoughts that are angry, or sad, or grouchy, then your body feels awful, too. That doesn't help you get better. Remember the story of changing sad cells into happy cells? (Go back and check if you don't — it's on page 33)

When you need chemotherapy, shots, and other treatments that are not fun at all, you might hate those treatments. Hate is a strong emotion that can affect your body in a negative way. Hating your medications or believing that they will hurt you can make you feel worse, too.

Let me tell you about Liliana, who had horrible pain for four days. She hid under the covers and moaned because she felt so awful.

She had a toothache and a great deal of pain in her jaw. The doctors did every test they could do, to try and figure out why she had this pain, but they couldn't find any reason at all. Liliana let me tap with her to see if it would help her feel a little better.

I asked her what she felt. Liliana said that she was mad at the doctor who gave her medications that made her feel really horrible. She believed the meds were harming her. That was a big problem.

Liliana didn't understand that sometimes the medications had to be strong in order to get way down deep where her body was sick. She also didn't understand that her angry thoughts were making the pain bigger than it had to be.

This is what we said as we tapped. Why don't you tap along with us and see how we made the pain smaller and smaller until it finally disappeared?

ROUND 1

Tap on the Karate Chop point and say:

Even though the pain is so BIG, I'm a great kid.

Even though it hurts so much, I'm a wonderful kid.

Even though I hate this pain and I want it to go away but it won't, I'm a great kid.

Eyebrow: I'm mad at my doctor.

Side of the Eye: My doctor is giving me medications that make me feel really, really awful.

Under the Eye: My doctor is hurting me with these horrible meds.

Under the Nose: I hate them. I don't want to take those bad meds.

Chin: I hate them. They make me feel so horrible.

Collarbone: I hate them. I don't want to take them.

Under the Arm: I fight everyone so I don't have to take the bad meds.

Top of the Head: I feel horrible because they make me take them anyway.

ROUND 2

Eyebrow: These horrible meds make me feel awful.

Side of the Eye: They make me feel sick.

Under the Eye: I throw up. I hate that.

Under the Nose: I don't want to take these meds.

Chin: They make me feel awful.

Collarbone: They're supposed to help me but I feel worse.

Under the Arm: I feel sick. I feel like throwing up.

Top of the Head: They harm me.

ROUND 3

Eyebrow: But the doctor is doing what he/she has learned to do — give me meds.

Side of the Eye: The doctor doesn't want me to feel terrible, he/she wants me to get better.

Under the Eye: I'm getting the drugs that my doctor feels are best for me.

Under the Nose: The doctor gives me the meds he/she has learned to give me.

Chin: The doctor spent many years learning about what to do to make me well, and, he/she gives me the meds that he/she knows.

Collarbone: I know I'm mad because the meds make me feel awful, but the doctor isn't trying to hurt me.

Under the Arm: My doctor wants me to get better so he/she gives me the meds he/she has learned to use.

Top of the Head: Instead of being mad at my doctor, I can tap so I feel better.

ROUND 4

Eyebrow: I'm not mad at the doctor anymore but I still believe that the meds hurt me.

Side of the Eye: I feel like the meds are damaging me.

Under the Eye: Those meds are really terrible.

Under the Nose: Those meds make me feel dizzy and sick to my stomach and then I throw up.

Chin: I'm so mad at those meds for making me feel awful.

Collarbone: The madder I am, the worse I feel.

Under the Arm: It hurts to be so mad at the meds.

Top of the Head: I feel pain because I'm so mad at the terrible meds.

ROUND 5

Eyebrow: I want to feel better, and not be mad at my meds.

Side of the Eye: The meds aren't trying to hurt me.

Under the Eye: They are just doing their job — like the doctor is.

Under the Nose: My meds don't want to be awful.

Chin: They want to be good.

Collarbone: They want to help me get better.

Under the Arm: I'd like them to help me.

Top of the Head: I don't want them to make me feel awful.

ROUND 6

Eyebrow: I want the meds to treat me well.

Side of the Eye: I want them to help me get better.

Under the Eye: I don't want them to make me feel sick.

Under the Nose: I want my meds to be good meds.

Chin: I want them to do their job without harming me.

Collarbone: What would happen if I didn't hate my meds?

Under the Arm: I might feel better. I could do something to make this work better too.

Top of the Head: I choose to stop hating my meds and let them help me instead.

ROUND 7

Eyebrow: I could send my meds a blessing instead.

Side of the Eye: I bless them for doing their job nicely.

Under the Eye: I surround the meds with love and a special colored light too. (What color do you choose?)

Under the Nose: I can make my meds into a magic healing potion.

Chin: A magic healing potion that heals my body.

Collarbone: A magic healing potion that gets rid of the sick parts.

Under the Arm: I like having a magic healing potion to help me get better. Anything is possible when you have a magic healing potion.

Top of the Head: I make my meds into a magic healing potion and I surround them with beautiful colored light. (Imagine whatever color you would like.)

ROUND 8

Eyebrow: I ask my body to let the meds do their job as if they were a magic healing potion.

Side of the Eye: My body knows how to let that happen and keep me feeling good.

Under the Eye: My body and my magic healing potion work together so I feel better.

Under the Nose: I like that my body and my meds are on the same team.

Chin: They work together so I feel better. That makes me feel good.

Collarbone: Working together feels so much better than hating my meds.

Under the Arm: I feel better already now that I don't hate my meds. I know that they are my magic healing potion and they are helping me to get better.

Top of the Head: I'm a good kid and I want to feel good.

ROUND 9

Eyebrow: I thank my meds because their job is to help me get better.

Side of the Eye: I imagine my meds surrounded by beautiful colored light and love that protects the meds and protects me from their nasty effects.

Under the Eye: My meds don't have to attack me and hurt me.

Under the Nose: My meds can do what they are supposed to – get rid of my illness – but leave the rest of me okay.

Chin: The colored light surrounds my meds and protects me from their nasty effects.

Collarbone: I'm really powerful. I can tell my meds to behave.

Under the Arm: I tell them to be a magic healing potion.

Top of the Head: I tell my meds to behave and to treat me well. I tell my meds to take care of me and not harm me, because they are my magic healing potion now.

ROUND 10

Eyebrow: I surround my meds with the colored light so that they can't hurt me.
Side of the Eye: I have magic healing potion meds.
Under the Eye: They are good meds, not bad meds.
Under the Nose: My meds are a magic healing potion that helps me to get better.
Chin: It makes me very powerful to tell my meds how to behave.
Collarbone: I tell my meds to help me get better and I tell my body to heal.
Under the Arm: This makes me powerful and ready to feel good.
Top of the Head: I like that I can talk to my body and my meds. It makes me powerful.

ROUND 11

Eyebrow: I have the power to choose to feel good.
Side of the Eye: I talk to my body. I talk to all of me. I tell my body to be calm.
Under the Eye: I talk to my meds. I tell them to be gentle with me.
Under the Nose: I tell my body and the meds to work together so I can feel better.
Chin: I know that my magic healing potion meds help me to get better.
Collarbone: I choose to have good meds, not bad meds, because I want to get better.
Under the Arm: I tap to feel better. I choose to get better.
Top of the Head: That makes me very powerful. And it helps me get better, too. Whoohoo!

LILIANA'S SORE TOOTH THAT WENT AWAY

Liliana hated her meds so much that her tooth hurt. The doctors couldn't figure what was making her tooth hurt so much. But when we tapped away the feelings that her meds were hurting her, and tapped away how much she hated them, she relaxed and her pain went away!

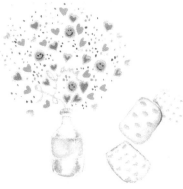

Pay attention to what you think about your meds. It could make a difference in how your body reacts to them. Send your meds love and bless them. Ask your meds to help you, not hurt you. You may find that you feel better and better.

Remember not to blame yourself if you feel awful or think negative thoughts. It's part of being human. What is important is to know that what you think and feel can make yourself feel worse or better. The best part is that you can choose how you think and feel. Tapping helps you feel good and think happy thoughts, rather than feeling awful, mad and sad. Which do you prefer?

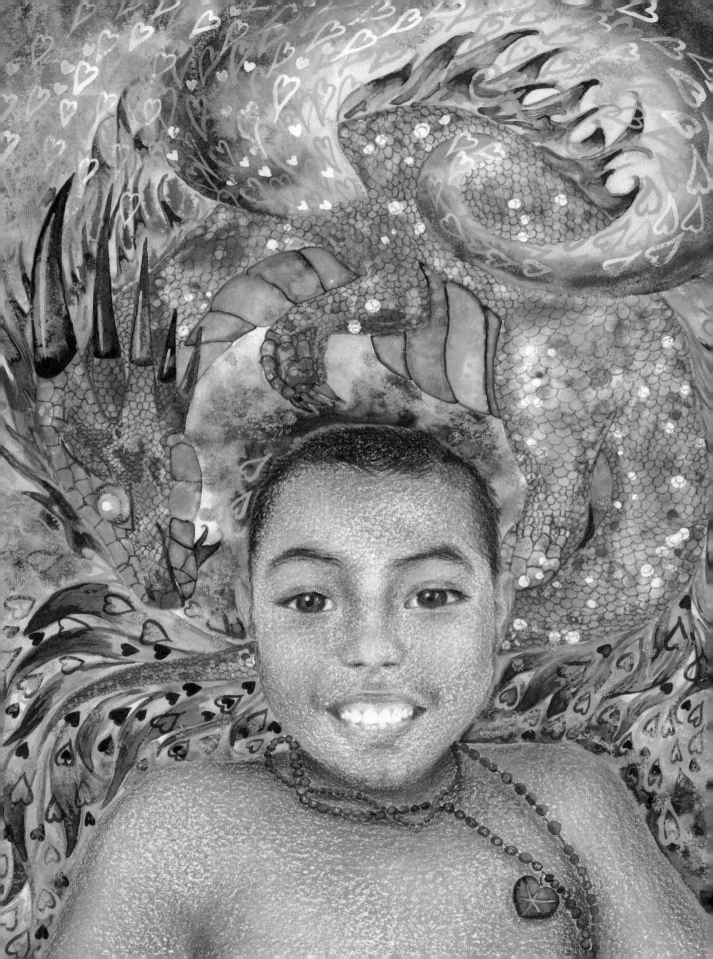

DIEGO AND THE DRAGON WITH FLAMES OF LOVE

*D*iego was really excited because he was finishing his two years of cancer treatments. He had big plans to be a graffiti style painter, except that he started to feel sick — he had a fever and he felt really tired.

When Diego went to what should have been his last appointment, his Doctor told him that he had had a relapse and would have to begin his treatments all over again. He couldn't imagine doing another two years of treatments.

Diego wasn't happy about it at all. In fact, he was very sad and didn't want to do anything. After two years of treatments, he thought he was done with hospitals but now he wasn't. It made him feel depressed. On top of it, he had a fever too.

What would you do if you were told you had had a relapse? How would you feel? Would you give up? Or would you do what Diego later did — get powerful and choose to get better again? Read on and see how that happened.

TappyBear and I came to visit Diego. Diego loved to tap with us because it always made him feel better, more relaxed and positive. I also helped him understand how his thoughts and feelings affected his body. That helped him make better decisions and allowed him to choose to be happy and do whatever it took to get better. Diego would tell me how it felt in his body when he tapped, and that helped us come up with Tapping statements that would work the best for him.

I asked Diego what animal made him feel strong. He said it was a dragon. The dragon then became his *'power animal.'* Do you know what a power animal is? No? Well, a power animal is any animal that, when you think of it, makes you feel stronger and more powerful. It can be any animal. Diego's is the dragon. Yours can be anything — maybe a tiger, a dog, a bear, a horse, a scorpion or even a cat or bunny!

Tap along to see how Diego used his power animal to feel better. You can use Diego's words and the power from his power animal or you can use your own power animal. Just say the name of your power animal every time the story says 'dragon' and instead of 'flames of love', put in what YOUR power animal does to make you strong — for example, roar, bark, stand tall, run like the wind, or anything else!

ROUND 1
Tap on the Karate Chop point and say:
Even though I don't want to be sick anymore, I'm a super great kid.
Even though the doctor told me I have to have more treatments, I'm a good kid.
Even though I don't want more treatments and I want to be done with hospitals, I am a great kid.

Eyebrow: I don't want to feel awful anymore.
Side of the Eye: I don't want to be sick.
Under the Eye: I have a nasty fever.

Under the Nose: I don't want to take more medicine. Yuck!

Chin: I want to play and have fun.

Collarbone: I want to spend time with my friends.

Under the Arm: I feel so sad.

Top of the Head: This is NO FUN!

This is the point where you choose your power animal. I asked Diego to keep his power animal, the *dragon*, in his mind as we continued to tap. Keep your power animal in your mind too.

ROUND 2

Eyebrow: I have a dragon. He is really powerful!

Side of the Eye: I have a powerful dragon to help me feel better.

Under the Eye: I have a friendly, helpful dragon.

Under the Nose: He wants me to get better and he is very strong.

Chin: When I think of him I feel stronger.

Collarbone: He is so powerful and breathes out fire.

Under the Arm: This fire is special.

Top of the Head: It is made of love.

ROUND 3

Eyebrow: The dragon has flames of love.

Side of the Eye: These flames of love are so beautiful.

Under the Eye: The flames of love are so strong and powerful.

Under the Nose: I feel how powerful they are; how powerful love is.

Chin: The flames of love make my body feel strong and powerful.

Collarbone: Love is the most powerful force there is.

Under the Arm: Love helps my body feel better.

Top of the Head: The flames of love make me feel happy and full of power.

ROUND 4

Eyebrow: I like being strong and I want to help my body feel better.

Side of the Eye: I ask my dragon with flames of love to come help me any time I want.

Under the Eye: Flames of love come from my dragon.

Under the Nose: This dragon is part of my power.

Chin: The flames of love get rid of all that is not good for me.

Collarbone: The flames of love get rid of all the nasty stuff.

Under the Arm: The flames of love heal the places in me that are hurt.

Top of the Head: The flames of love warm me, hug me and love me.

ROUND 5

Eyebrow: I feel so good when the flames of love protect me from all harm.

Side of the Eye: The flames of love from my dragon are my friends.

Under the Eye: My body knows that, and it makes my body feel better.

Under the Nose: My body is enveloped in flames of love. I love that. I love my dragon with flames of love.

Chin: The flames of love transform the places in me that are not healthy.

Collarbone: The flames of love change the horrible into good.

Under the Arm: The flames of love take the sickness out of my cells and make them better.

Top of the Head: The flames of love surround my sadness and any parts that are sick and makes them feel so loved, so hugged, and so beautiful, that they get better.

ROUND 6

Eyebrow: Love is so healing. Love helps me get better.

Side of the Eye: I love that the flames of love grow inside of me.

Under the Eye: They grow inside the parts of me that are sick.

Under the Nose: Love makes me feel good, hugged, cared for and loved.

Chin: That heals my heart and lets my body get better too.

Collarbone: Love is so powerful, just like my dragon with flames of love.

Under the Arm: When I love, I am powerful too. My body feels powerful.

Top of the Head: Love makes my body powerful so I can get better.

The flames of love coming out of the *dragon* made Diego feel loved and cared for.

The flames of love made his body feel strong. His fever went away. He decided he wanted to get better again. He had the power to choose to be happy and enjoy each day. Diego used EFT every day, along with his *dragon* with flames of love to help him get better and better. You can, too!

When you feel awful or get bad news, you too can tap with your *power animal* to feel better. Imagine the animal that makes you feel strong and powerful, helping you and making you strong. Tap with your *power animal* every day. You can ask it to always be there to help you. Together you will be very powerful. You make a great team!

This story about Diego's power animal, the *dragon*, is how the title of this book, "The Dragon with Flames of Love," came into being. Thank you, Diego.

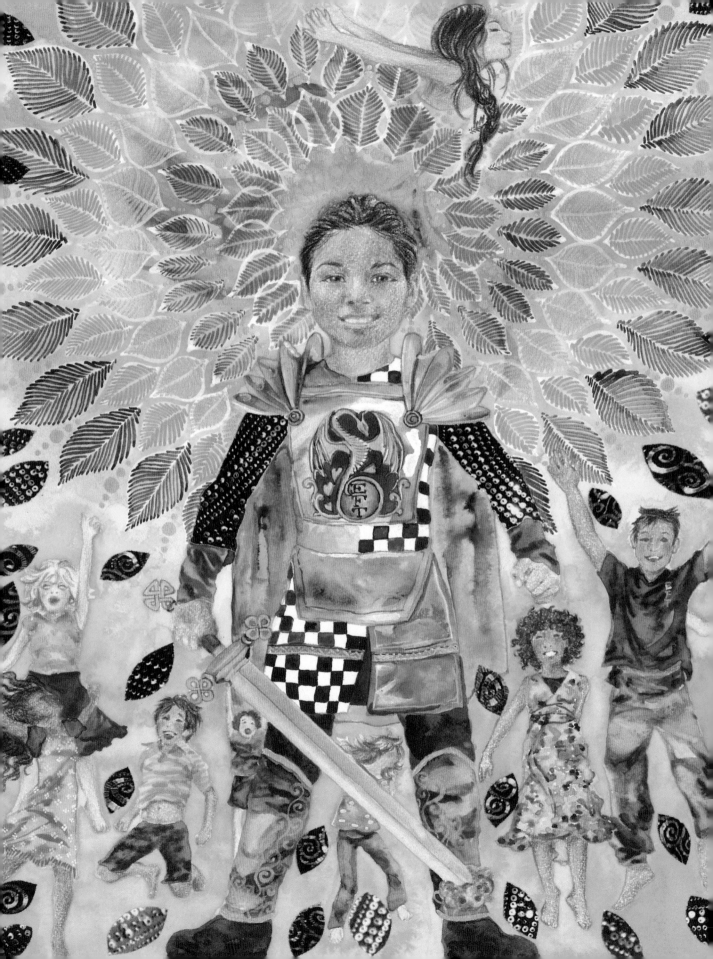

RODOLFO, AN EFT CHAMPION

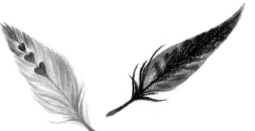

Eleven-year old Rodolfo is an EFT champion. He didn't start out being a champion. Actually, he was quite critical. (Someone who is critical is always finding something wrong, or finding fault.) Rodolfo agreed that he was even very critical of himself. He was constantly upset with himself for not doing things perfectly. He was even critical with himself for not healing quickly enough. There was always something about himself or his family that he didn't think was good enough. It's really hard to be perfect all the time.

Since he didn't like being so self-critical, Rodolfo and I looked for ways for him to be nicer to himself. We also looked at how emotions can affect different parts of our bodies.

If you are usually happy and cheerful, this will affect your body in a good way, making it feel better. If you are often angry and grumpy, then this will make your body upset too.

Different parts of the body, such as the heart, kidney, liver, arms, legs and back, each do different jobs. It is interesting to know that some emotions or feelings connect more strongly with certain body parts.

If you feel 'put-down' or criticized by other people, or if you are very critical of yourself, then theses emotions tend to have a stronger effect on the kidneys. Just like Rodolfo. He was super critical of himself all the time and the part of his body that was unhealthy was his right kidney. He had a tumor there. It was painful — just like being critical of himself all the time was painful, too.

Pay attention and you'll recognize if you are critical or mean to yourself. Think about these questions:

♥ Are you critical of yourself?

♥ Where are you most critical — at school, at home or someplace else?

♥ Why? Is it because of the way you look, or because there's something you don't do well?

Tap along with us so that you, too, can change from being critical of yourself to being nice to yourself.

ROUND 1

Tap on the Karate Chop point and say:

Even though I'm so critical of myself, I'm a great kid.

Even though I'm so hard on myself, I'm a great kid.

Even though I blame myself for doing things badly, I'm a loveable kid.

Eyebrow: I'm so critical of myself.

Side of the Eye: I always tell myself I am bad, or I've done something poorly.

Under the Eye: I put myself down.

Under the Nose: I am hard on myself, just like my tumor.

Chin: I'm really hard on myself.

Collarbone: I tell myself all the time how bad I am.

Under the Arm: I tell myself I'm not good enough.

Top of the Head: And I believe it.

ROUND 2

Eyebrow: I criticize others, too.

Side of the Eye: I'm hard on them, too.

Under the Eye: I tell them they're not good enough.

Under the Nose: I get mad at them.

Chin: Then my family gets mad at me.

Collarbone: My family criticizes me, too.

Under the Arm: They are hard on me.

Top of the Head: All that ugly criticism. It feels so awful. It feels so hard.

ROUND 3

Eyebrow: I had so many hard and mean thoughts.

Side of the Eye: I had hard, mean thoughts every day.

Under the Eye: This hard tumor in my kidney is just like my hard thoughts.

Under the Nose: My body made a hard tumor to store all that criticism.

Chin: I was so mean to myself that my body looked for a place to hide all that meanness and hardness.

Collarbone: It found a place to hide that criticism, in the tumor in my kidney.

Under the Arm: My body tried to take that criticism and pack it all into one small place.

Top of the Head: My body tried to defend me by storing all that criticism in my tumor.

ROUND 4

Eyebrow: My body tried to hide it so that it wouldn't hurt me so much.

Side of the Eye: Being mean to myself really hurts. Being mean to others hurts too.

Under the Eye: I felt hurt when other people didn't like what I said or did.

Under the Nose: It hurts when people say bad things about me, even if I'm used to talking about myself that way.

Chin: I am cruel to myself sometimes.

Collarbone: I don't even know why I'm so mean to myself.

Under the Arm: I can be so mean to my family too.

Top of the Head: I don't like being critical of myself and my family.

ROUND 5

Eyebrow: I'm tired of being mean to myself.

Side of the Eye: I can change. It's my choice. I can choose to be nicer to myself instead.

Under the Eye: I'll start by looking for something that I did well.

Under the Nose: I'm not used to being nice to myself, but I'll practice every day.

Chin: I can find good things about myself if I try and then comment on them.

Collarbone: For example, I'm actually a good kid so I can stop being mean to myself.

Under the Arm: I choose to be kinder to myself even if I make a mistake.

Top of the Head: This may take some practice and it may even take a long time, but it will feel good to be nice to myself.

ROUND 6

Eyebrow: I choose to look at the good things in me.

Side of the Eye: I choose to be nice to myself.

Under the Eye: I'm a great kid and I'm talented.

Under the Nose: I can be nice to my family too.

Chin: I choose to say nice things about myself and others.

Collarbone: I choose to praise myself when I do well.

Under the Arm: I am worthy. Actually, I'm an amazing kid.

Top of the Head: I say nice things to myself and nice things to others. I can choose to look at the good things.

Rodolfo felt much better because he had made a choice to be nicer to himself. He would like you to do the same.

THE YELLOW SWORD

When it was time to have surgery to remove the tumor, Rodolfo was afraid, but he knew he could tap away all of those fears. Tap along now so you can feel strong if you have a tumor, or if you have to have surgery too.

I asked Rodolfo to imagine what his tumor looked like. Rodolfo said it was about the size of a grapefruit and that the tumor cells were inside of that grapefruit.

Then I asked Rodolfo, "If you imagine doing whatever you need to, in order to remove that tumor, what would you do?" He said, "Cut it out with a sword." Of course, it was a magic sword — a magic yellow sword. If you had a magic sword, what would it look like? What color would it be? And what would you use it for?

Rodolfo tapped while imagining using his magic yellow sword to get rid of the tumor. Then he tapped while imagining the doctors taking out the tumor so he could be completely healed. Tap along with Rodolfo now.

ROUND 7

Tap on the Karate Chop point and say:
Even though I have this ugly tumor inside of me, I'm a wonderful kid.
Even though I don't like this ugly tumor that looks like a grapefruit, I'm a great kid.
Even though I want to get rid of this grapefruit-size tumor, I'm an amazing kid.

Eyebrow: I have a magic sword. It makes me powerful.
Side of the Eye: My powerful magic sword gives me the strength to take out all the bad words I have said to myself.
Under the Eye: My magic yellow sword cuts out all the bad, mean words I've said about myself.
Under the Nose: All those mean words stored in my tumor can be cut into little pieces and made to disappear — PUFF!! Just like that.
Chin: My magic sword cuts those mean words into little bits.
Collarbone: My magic sword cuts all the hard thoughts I had about myself into little pieces.
Under the Arm: My body gets rid of them. PUFF! They're gone.
Top of the Head: I don't need them anymore. I'm going to be nice to myself now.

ROUND 8

Eyebrow: My magic sword gets rid of all the mean things I said to others, too.
Side of the Eye: I cut out all the bad and mean things I said and get rid of them.
Under the Eye: My magic sword cuts out any leftover mean words so they can be taken out and disappear. They aren't needed anymore.
Under the Nose: Even the tiniest mean thought or feeling gets cut out.
Chin: My magic sword takes out all the mean words and leaves room for good words.
Collarbone: It is safe for me to be nice to myself. I'm ready for kind and loving words to fill up all the space left by the mean words that are now gone.
Under the Arm: I use my sword to cut that tumor into tiny pieces too. Here it goes: cut, cut, cut. All that's left are tiny pieces.
Top of the Head: My body gently and safely removes all those pieces too.

Roldolfo cut out all the bad 'energy' of his words and thoughts that was stored in that tumor. He imagined cutting the tumor into little pieces with his magic sword. Now he was ready for the doctors to take out the physical tumor too. It, too, wasn't needed anymore. Rodolfo likes angels, so he asked that some angels come to protect him and take care of the doctors and nurses too.

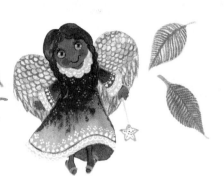

ROUND 9

Eyebrow: Before the surgery, I'm smiling and laughing with the nurses and doctors.
Side of the Eye: They treat me really well.
Under the Eye: They take care of me.
Under the Nose: I go to sleep without worries.
Chin: I know the surgeon is doing his best work.
Collarbone: I ask that five angels be there with me to take care of me and the doctors and nurses. One for each of us — even one for my tumor.
Under the Arm: I trust that everything will come out just fine. I trust that my tumor can be taken out easily.
Top of the Head: I send my tumor a blessing for holding all my criticism and tell it that it doesn't have to do that anymore.

ROUND 10

Eyebrow: My sword gets me ready for the surgery too.
Side of the Eye: I take out all the bad energy in the tumor with my sword.
Under the Eye: The doctors will take out the physical part of that tumor.
Under the Nose: It's okay to have the doctors help me take out this tumor that holds my mean thoughts.
Chin: The doctors cut out the tumor and with it, all the cells that carry my mean thoughts.
Collarbone: The doctors carefully take out the tumor, and that automatically removes the place where I store the mean old thoughts, too.
Under the Arm: We take out where I stored the mean stuff. It means I get to start over again without criticizing myself.
Top of the Head: It means I can start telling myself good things to fill up the empty space that's left. It means I can love myself.

Rodolfo was ready for the surgery. He went in with a positive attitude, feeling sure that everything was going to go well. And it did!

After the surgery, Rodolfo tapped to make sure he stayed positive and didn't go back to saying mean things to himself. You can do that too. Tap a little every day so that you can keep saying good things to yourself.

ROUND 11

Tap on the Karate Chop point and say:

Even though I used to be mean to myself a lot, I don't have to do that anymore.

Even though I used to be mean and critical of myself, I'm free of that now. I'm free to love myself as I should.

Even though I used to say nasty things about myself, I now say nice things about myself.

Eyebrow: I'm an awesome kid and I'm kind to myself.

Side of the Eye: I don't take things personally.

Under the Eye: I know when something is about me and when it isn't.

Under the Nose: I am a good kid, not bad.

Chin: I tell myself what a good kid I am, and then I do good things, too.

Collarbone: I don't have to be critical of myself. I don't have to have others be critical of me either.

Under the Arm: Instead of criticizing others, I compliment them on their good traits.

Top of the Head: I say nice things about myself too, because I love myself.

ROUND 12

Eyebrow: I'm nice to myself because I'm a good kid.

Side of the Eye: I like being nice to myself because it makes me happy.

Under the Eye: Being nice to myself let's me be nice to others, too.

Under the Nose: Then everyone feels good. I like that.

Chin: I want everyone to feel good and to know that deep inside they are good.

Collarbone: I look for the good things inside me. I look for the good things in others. It makes me feel so good, so happy.

Under the Arm: I love how it makes me feel good. I love how it makes others feel good too.

Top of the Head: Loving myself feels so good and makes my body feel so good, too.

Rodolfo kept tapping so that he would stay nice to himself. You can do the same. And look at what else Rodolfo did!

RODOLFO IS AN EFT CHAMPION

Wow! Rodolfo is a young man who taps every day — and not only that. Because he recognizes how great he feels when he does EFT, he took it upon himself to teach his family and friends. He taps every day with his parents. He taught his younger sister and brother, his aunts and uncles, his cousins and his best friends. Two of his friends come over every day after school and they tap together. He had promised to tap twice a day so he would be kind to himself, and not critical — but he went way beyond that.

When I see him, I realize how well he is doing. He looks fabulous. He has a full head of hair, has grown taller, and has the most incredible smile. But beyond all of that, the most obvious thing you notice is the feeling of peace around him. You can see it in his eyes. That's why Rodolfo is an EFT Champion.

You can be an EFT Champion too! Tap every day and share Tapping with everyone you love so they can benefit from it too.

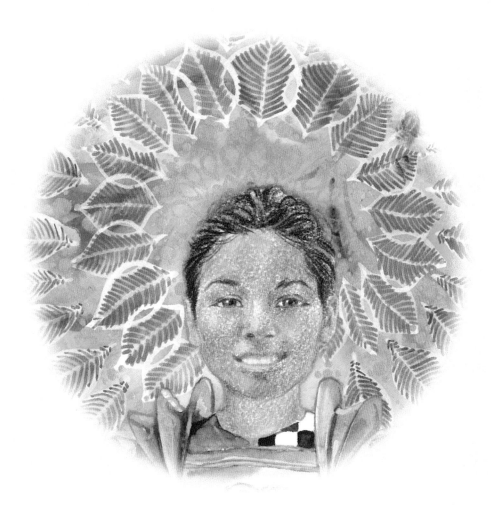

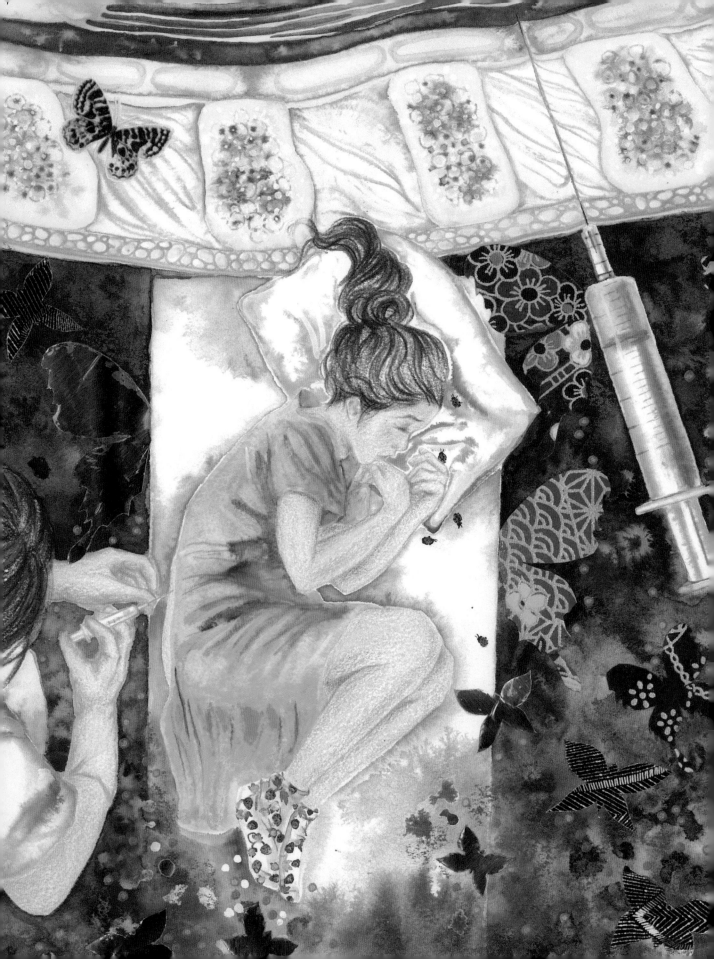

SPINAL TAP:
BIG NEEDLE, LITTLE HURT

NOTE TO PARENTS:

A spinal tap is one of the treatments that children fight against the most, because of the positioning and the pain that can be associated with it. Let's look at how we can make this treatment as gentle and painless as possible.

*F*irst of all, teaching your child about what is going to happen allows him or her to participate in making the experience better. If your child is tense and frightened, the procedure is more painful. When they are calm, many children go through the whole process as if it were a little pinprick.

Secondly, let's teach your child a few tricks. Show your child your fist when it is closed tightly and tap on it to show how hard it is. Say that is how your back is when it is tense. Then make a closed hand but let it be relaxed. Tap on it to show how it is relaxed and pliable. That is how your back is when you are relaxed. When you are relaxed it is easier for the needle to go in.

How do you get your body to relax? Breathing deeply helps calm the body and relax the back. Inhale deeply and let the shoulders and back droop as if you were a rag doll. Do this several times. Doing this will help your child immensely to understand how he or she can affect this procedure in a positive way.

Thirdly, visualize and tap about all the fears and anxieties your child has regarding this treatment. This will help your child release his or her fear of each step before he or she actually has the injection. Here's the procedure: your child will visualize the whole procedure from beginning to end and tap away any anxieties step by step, until he or she can imagine going through the treatment from start to finish calmly. If the child can imagine it and see it in his or her mind's eye first, it is much easier to go through the procedure afterwards.

For example: Ask your child to imagine that they are going to have a spinal tap. Tap until all fears are gone. Have your child imagine walking into the treatment room. Tap until your child is calm again. Have your child imagine getting on the treatment table. Tap away any fears. Have your child imagine the doctor coming in. Tap away any fears. Have your child imagine the doctor cleaning his or her back with that cold sterilizing liquid. Tap away any fears. Have your child imagine the doctor with the needle. Tap away any fears. Have your child imagine the actual injection. Tap away any fears. Have your child imagine finishing the injection and walking back to the bed. Tap away any fears or pain. Then, have your child review the whole treatment again, while tapping until there is no fear or any thoughts of pain while visualizing the entire process.

This visualization is a very important step because it prepares your child emotionally, mentally and physically for what is going to happen. This means there won't be any shock, fear or surprises when it actually does happen. Everything will be just as they imagined it, and that will help them to be calm and feel in control of the situation.

In many cases, feelings of fear, anxiety or trauma result from a sensation of helplessness. Not knowing what is going to happen to us, or feeling that we are not able to do anything about it, can be very scary — both for adults and children! Visualizing and Tapping are two fantastic tools that we can use to empower ourselves, helping us feel calm and in control. This makes it possible for us to relax, even in potentially difficult or stressful situations.

Now, the fourth step is to tap with your child during the actual procedure, in order to keep your child and yourself calm. Because of the restricted space in most treatment rooms and the position of the body, it may be easier if you — the parent — tap on your child. Tap on the points that you can reach, which may be only the point on the top of the head or the Karate Chop point. That's okay. Tap there continually during the entire process. Remind your child to breathe deeply and to try and visualize something that, for them, is relaxing and happy — for example, a green field and blue sky, the beach, a favorite toy, a special friend, their last birthday party or summer holiday, anything they like.

Finally, tap after the treatment is over, so that any pain and trauma experienced can be released immediately. With Tapping, children normally relax and release the pain within 2-3 minutes and many fall asleep calmly. This Tapping allows the body to forget the trauma too.

Some real-life examples: Rodolfo found that with Tapping, his pain was five times less than other times he had a spinal injection. Rodrigo used to receive tranquilizers in order for the doctors to be able to come near him. But after Tapping, he would allow them to give him the spinal tap. Sergio used to dread having a spinal tap, but now it is part of the routine. Janeth calmly walks in and gets her spinal tap without fuss or worry now, thanks to Tapping.

In this story, Brenda was afraid of having a spinal tap. Really afraid. I taught her how to do Tapping to make it easier. This Tapping story is based on her experience. Brenda used a power animal, just like Diego did in "The Dragon with Flames of Love." You can go back and review that story if you have forgotten how to use a power animal. Brenda's power animal is a dolphin, because it makes her feel free.

0-10 SCALE

You can use a scale to determine how much pain or fear is being felt. The scale is a simple number scale from 0-10, where 0 is no fear or pain and 10 is the maximum emotion or pain felt. Every number in between is an intermediate value. If your child is too young to answer with a number, just have your child stretch out his or her hands to show how big it is. Closed hands means 0 and completely out-stretched means 10.

Ask how much pain or fear the child is feeling. It is a subjective answer, but it can be used

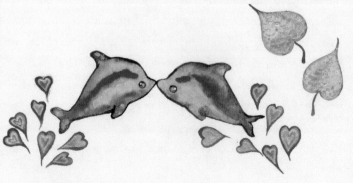

periodically throughout the Tapping to help the child realize how much the pain or fear is reducing. This helps the child feel better. Sometimes the number goes up before it comes down, and that's okay too. If the number isn't changing at all, then different words need to be used or you may need to find out what else is wrong.

BRENDA'S BIG FEAR

Brenda tapped with me to prepare for a spinal tap. First, I had her imagine that she was going to have the treatment. She answered the following questions: What do you feel? Her answer was "Afraid." How BIG is that fear? On a scale of 0-10 Brenda's answer was a 9. Then she tapped, saying the following sentences. You can do it, too.

ROUND 1

Tap on the Karate Chop point and say:
Even though I'm afraid of having a spinal tap because it hurts so much, I'm a good kid.
Even though I don't want to have a needle in my back because it scares me, I'm a great kid.
Even though I am afraid that it will hurt when they put a needle in my back, I'm a fabulous kid.

Eyebrow: I imagine myself having a spinal tap.
Side of the Eye: I imagine what I feel.
Under the Eye: I feel scared. (Or name whatever emotion comes up.)
Under the Nose: I am afraid it will hurt.
Chin: It hurt in the past.
Collarbone: I'm sure it will hurt again.
Under the Arm: I don't like to be poked in the back.
Top of the Head: The nurse puts a cream on my back but it still hurts.

ROUND 2

Eyebrow: I'm afraid. This fear is so big.
Side of the Eye: It hurts already and I haven't even gone into the treatment room.
Under the Eye: I worry about how much it will hurt.
Under the Nose: I don't want to hurt.
Chin: I am afraid.
Collarbone: I am afraid of going in there. It hurts when they poke me in the back.
Under the Arm: I don't like it. I'm scared. I don't like how it hurts.
Top of the Head: I'm so afraid of this.

ROUND 3

Eyebrow: My legs go numb.

Side of the Eye: My back hurts.

Under the Eye: It is uncomfortable to be all scrunched over.

Under the Nose: My body aches from sitting like that.

Chin: I don't want to be poked.

Collarbone: It scares me so much.

Under the Arm: I'm afraid it will hurt.

Top of the Head: That is my biggest fear — that it will hurt.

On the scale of 0-10, Brenda's fear was now down to a 6.

I had Brenda imagine her fear as if it were a color. The color symbolically represented the pain. Your child can choose whatever color comes into his or her mind.

ROUND 4

Eyebrow: That big fear is black. (Put in the color that your child imagines.)

Side of the Eye: That ugly black in my back.

Under the Eye: That black is so BIG.

Under the Nose: It is as BIG as my fear.

Chin: That black makes me tense.

Collarbone: That black makes me tight.

Under the Arm: That big black fear of mine.

Top of the Head: It is so BIG. That big, ugly black.

ROUND 5

Eyebrow: I don't have to have that black.

Side of the Eye: I can take the ugly black fear and throw it away.

Under the Eye: I throw all the black in the trash.

Under the Nose: I throw all of the black fear in the trash.

Chin: That black can't stay if I don't let it.

Collarbone: I take the black and throw it out.

Under the Arm: With it the fear goes, too.

Top of the Head: All the fear and black go in the trash.

I asked Brenda to imagine going into the treatment room again. How big is the fear now? For Brenda it was a 4. If your child still feels the fear, go back and tap again until the fear is gone. It's perfectly normal to do many rounds of Tapping until a fear is gone. The important thing is to get rid of it completely.

Keep checking about the number and the color to see if they change as you go. Usually, as you keep tapping the number goes down and down until it reaches zero and is gone; the color changes to a less ugly/fearful color and then to more happy, pretty colors with more positive associations for the child. Note: Do not suggest a number or color to your child. Let them decide on one themselves, even if they take a while to find it. Normally, the first number or color that pops into their head is the 'right' answer.

I checked with Brenda to see what the fear was about. Was she fearful of going into the room? Getting on the treatment table? Was it that cold liquid the doctor uses to clean her back? Is it the poking fingers on her back? Is it the needle itself? Or more than one of these things?

In Brenda's case the fear was of the needle. She thought it was enormous. We tapped to make that big, ugly, painful needle into one that was tiny and gentle.

ROUND 6

Eyebrow: That enormous needle. It scares me.

Side of the Eye: That enormous needle. I don't like it.

Under the Eye: I think that needle is enormous. It feels enormous.

Under the Nose: I'm afraid of that big needle.

Chin: That big needle hurts so much that I don't want a spinal tap.

Collarbone: I shake with fear because of that needle. I don't want to feel this fear.

Under the Arm: I want to find a way to get rid of this fear.

Top of the Head: I want to find a way to not be afraid of it.

ROUND 7

Eyebrow: I can use Tapping and the power of my imagination to change how I feel about that needle.

Side of the Eye: I think that needle is enormous but it actually isn't that big.

Under the Eye: I tap and imagine the big needle getting smaller and smaller, back to its true size.

Under the Nose: I take the enormous needle and I make it smaller and smaller. I have a magic remote control and I can make it as small as I want.

Chin: It is big in my mind, but it actually isn't so big in real life.

Collarbone: In fact, it's quite thin.

Under the Arm: I can deal with a thin needle. I can relax with a thin needle.

Top of the Head: I relax and it goes right in, to the perfect spot. I don't even feel it go in.

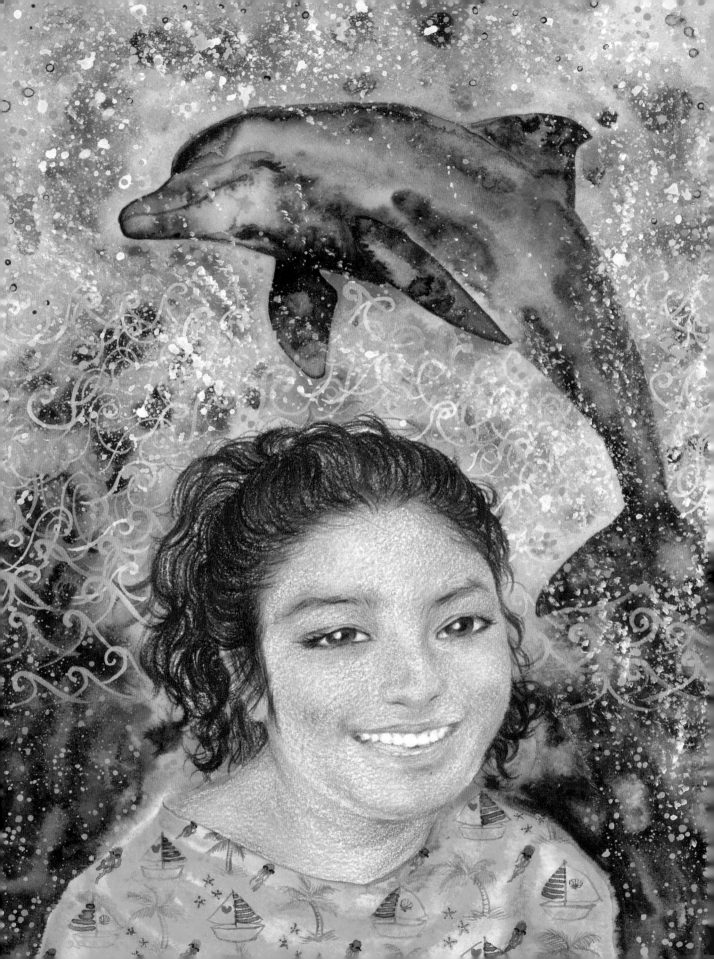

I asked Brenda what she thought about the needle now. She said it felt thinner and that made her believe it could go in easily. Her fear dropped to a 2. I decided to have Brenda bring in her power animal. Remember in Brenda's case it is the freedom-giving dolphin, but your child's power animal could be something completely different.

ROUND 8

Eyebrow: I take my power animal with me too.
Side of the Eye: I take my dolphin with me because I feel powerful then.
Under the Eye: The dolphin is so happy and free.
Under the Nose: The dolphin helps me to be as relaxed as if I were swimming in the sea.
Chin: The dolphin smiles at me and that makes me laugh.
Collarbone: The joy of the dolphin helps me be relaxed too.
Under the Arm: My dolphin reminds me that I can choose to be calm.
Top of the Head: My dolphin reminds me that it can always go better than I imagine.

Brenda's fear dropped to 0. She was now ready. How about you — are you ready? Is your child ready? If his or her fear is at 0, then congratulations! They are ready to have the treatment. Remember to tap with your child when you are in the treatment room. Maybe it is only possible to tap on their karate chop point or the top of their head or even some of the face points, but that is okay. Tap where you can, so that you both stay as calm as possible. If you don't feel calm, then tap some more until you do.

I helped Brenda feel even more confident by doing more tapping right before she went into the treatment room. Do what Brenda and I did. Visualize how you want the procedure to go. Then go have your treatment calmly. Remember to tap on your child or to help them tap themselves during the treatment.

ROUND 9

Even though I don't like to have a spinal tap, I am a great kid.
Even though I'm all tense now that I'm in the treatment room, I breathe and relax.
Even though I know it might hurt, I breathe deeply and relax.

Eyebrow: Sitting here makes me tense.
Side of the Eye: I worry it might be like before.
Under the Eye: But this is a different time so it can be better.
Under the Nose: I talk to my body and tell it to relax.
Chin: I breathe deeply and shake all the tension from my body.
Collarbone: I breathe deeply and get into the best position ever.

Under the Arm: I breathe deeply and calm myself.

Top of the Head: I want to be calm so everything goes well.

ROUND 10

Eyebrow: I am strong and powerful.

Side of the Eye: I'm a powerful kid who chooses to have this go well.

Under the Eye: I am strong and I have my power animal with me, too.

Under the Nose: I breathe deeply and my back muscles relax.

Chin: Breathing deeply keeps me from being tense.

Collarbone: Breathing deeply and Tapping keeps me from feeling pain.

Under the Arm: When my back muscles are relaxed the needle goes in easily.

Top of the Head: I am relaxed so it all happens as gently as possible.

ROUND 11

Eyebrow: I continue to breathe and my mom/dad taps on me.

Side of the Eye: I let the doctor get everything ready. I am calm.

Under the Eye: I let the doctor clean my back so everything is super clean.

Under the Nose: I breathe and hold still so everything goes well. I am calm.

Chin: I let that needle go directly to the perfect spot because I am calm.

Collarbone: The doctor quickly takes the sample.

Under the Arm: The doctor quickly puts in the meds and takes out the needle.

Top of the Head: I'm so glad it is done and now I can relax completely.

Once your treatment is over, go back to your bed; tap again so that anything that aches or hurts goes away. That's what Brenda did and she felt much better for it. There is no need for your body to hold onto any fear or pain after a treatment.

ROUND 12

Even though the doctor poked me in the back and it hurt a bit, I'm a great kid.

Even though my back is sore from that needle, I'm a wonderful kid.

Even though my back aches and I don't want to move, I love myself.

Eyebrow: I did better. It didn't hurt as much.

Side of the Eye: It still hurt some. I don't like that.

Under the Eye: I don't want to hurt at all.

Under the Nose: But it's over now, so I can relax.

Chin: I tell my back it is okay to let go of all the pain.

Collarbone: I tell my back to get rid of the pain.

Under the Arm: It's over now, so my back can relax.

Top of the Head: I let all the pain go.

ROUND 13

Eyebrow: I tell my body it is over and it can relax.

Side of the Eye: All the tightness in my back can go away.

Under the Eye: The pain can go away.

Under the Nose: I tell the pain it is all over and it can go.

Chin: The pain starts to slip away.

Collarbone: I feel my back relaxing.

Under the Arm: I feel better now.

Top of the Head: I take a deep breath.

ROUND 14

Eyebrow: Even the place where the needle poked my back relaxes.

Side of the Eye: It is like my back sighs and lets go of all the pain and tension.

Under the Eye: Even the spot where the needle poked me relaxes.

Under the Nose: I tell my body it is over now and it can forget what happened.

Chin: It is done and my body can forget it.

Collarbone: My back doesn't have to remember the pain.

Under the Arm: My back can let it go and relax.

Top of the Head: My whole body relaxes and I feel so calm.

ROUND 15

Eyebrow: I get better and better at doing this every time.

Side of the Eye: I breathe deeply and everything is better.

Under the Eye: I'm a great kid, strong and powerful.

Under the Nose: I am so powerful that I can do anything.

Chin: My back is strong and powerful too.

Collarbone: Together we can do anything.

Under the Arm: I'm a great kid, and I'm strong and powerful.

Top of the Head: I am so powerful that I can do anything.

ROUND 16

Eyebrow: The dolphin reminds me that I'm powerful.

Side of the Eye: Since I'm so powerful, I can send away anything that bothers me.

Under the Eye: The dolphin talks to me in that dolphin way and nods its head up and down telling me that yes I can feel good.

Under the Nose: The dolphin and I laugh together.

Chin: The dolphin is always there to remind me that I'm free to feel good.

Collarbone: I like feeling good, so I remind my body to feel good.

Under the Arm: My dolphin and I laugh and feel good.

Top of the Head: I like feeling good and so does my body.

Brenda relaxed completely. It was the best treatment she had had so far. She felt powerful because she didn't have to be afraid of a spinal tap and she could tap to feel better before, during and after. That gave her freedom, just like her power animal, the dolphin.

Just like Brenda, you can let go of the hurt and any aches or pains in your body. Then you can relax and fall asleep, waking up feeling like nothing happened. That is the power of Tapping and having your power animal with you. Call in the power animal that makes you feel strong and powerful so you can have better experiences with a spinal tap and any other treatment you find scary or difficult.

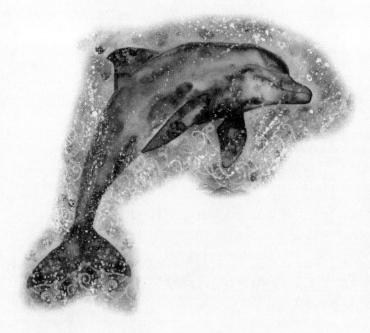

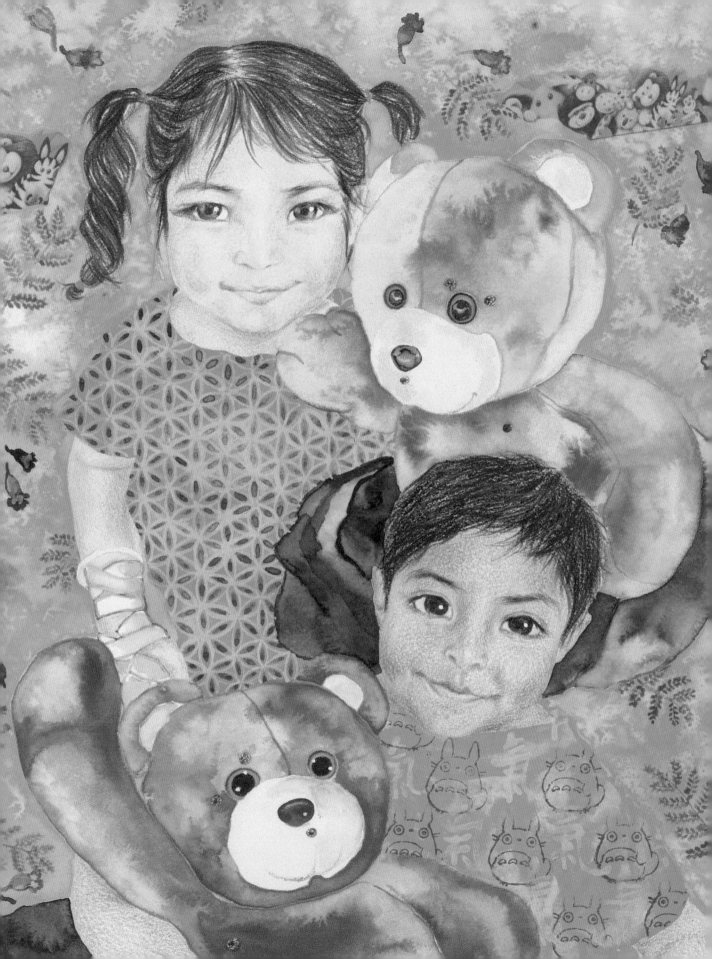

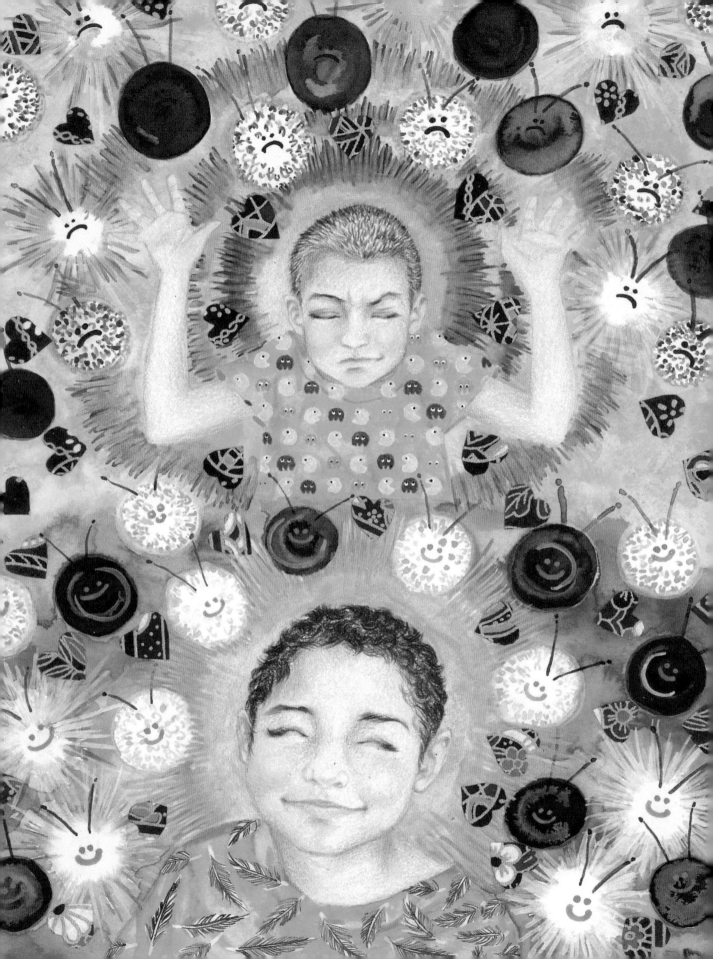

TAPPY CHAT WITH YOUR BLOOD CELLS

Kevin is an enthusiastic and cheerful young man. He also has leukemia. Sometimes when he feels down because of his treatments or because his defenses are low, he and I discuss how you can 'talk' to your body, to your cells, and to the parts of you that are ill or feel awful.

This has helped Kevin change the way he thinks about his illness. He feels very powerful to be able to talk to his body. He feels powerful because he can actively be involved in helping his body get better by continually sending happy, positive and uplifting messages about healing while he is Tapping.

How is it possible that you can 'talk' to your cells? First, let's look at how cells 'listen.' Cells have receptors on their surface. You can think of them like little antennae on the surface of the cell. They are 'listening' or responding to every signal that comes to them. These messages come from what you eat, from the environment around you (is it healthy or toxic, happy or sad?), from what you think and feel, and from other cells sharing what's going on in other parts of the body.

The antennae pick up all of these messages and send them inside your cells. The cells then make whatever substances are needed to answer those messages. If everything is negative, sad, toxic and horrible, the cells receive a message to create more chemicals in the body that make you feel even more negative and sad. When things are happy, playful and fun, the cells make more substances that make you feel even happier.

Don't worry if you feel sad sometimes or ugly things are happening around you. Cells manage really well — even in a bad situation. They will do their best to find a way to clean up the mess and make substances that heal them. They are programmed to do their best to heal, all the time. But sometimes they could use a little help from you. And you can help your cells by sending them good messages.

Doctors know that if you are happy and content, your immune system will get stronger and if you are sad all the time, it will get weaker. You can help your cells by sending them good messages, and by thinking good thoughts.

Actually choosing what you think lets you have a lot of control, kind of like a pilot directing where a plane will go. In this case, you send good messages to your cells. You can make a HUGE difference by changing first how you think and then, how you feel. Instead of being sad and unhappy about being sick, you can imagine how you want your body to get better. *The cells in your body will do their best to do exactly what you imagine them doing.* That makes you very powerful! You can sing, dance, laugh, smile, talk about fun things or talk directly to your cells and tell them how you'd like to feel. You can even send them a lot of love. How cool is that?

Thinking positive thoughts allows you, just like Kevin, to 'talk' to your cells and help them get better. Sometimes these little chats are just enough to tip the scale in your favor. That is really a good thing to do.

If you have problems with your blood, it is a good thing to know a little about what makes up the blood in your body so you can send a good message directly to your blood cells. That way you will know how to speak their language.

Kevin has leukemia or blood cancer, so we looked at the cells that make up blood.

The body has three types of blood cells: **red blood cells, white blood cells** and **platelets**. Each one has a special job to do.

♥ **Red blood cells** carry oxygen from the lungs to the tissues throughout the body. You can think of them like a big red dump truck carrying oxygen all around your body and delivering it exactly where it is needed. That's why breathing deeply is so important. When you breathe deeply, your red blood cells pick up more oxygen to carry into your body. That makes them feel good.

♥ **White blood cells** help fight infection. They are some of the body's warriors, which means they make up part of our defense system. There are several types of white blood cells. I'll mention some of their jobs.

Some white blood cells (neutrophils) are at the front line and they are the first to attack an invader. They throw a chemical substance at the invader and then engulf it or eat it.

A small number of the white blood cells in your body are like the 'Pacman' of your defenses. They form monocytes or macrophages that surround harmful bacteria and have chemical substances inside of them that destroy the bad guys.

Lymphocytes form the major part of your blood's defense system. The two main ones, B cells and T cells, work together. The B cells recognize the invading bad guys, and mark them. The T cells then get rid of the marked bad guys. These two working together are very important to being healthy. There are others that support them in this work, too.

A problem occurs when your own white blood cells get sick. They don't function right and they don't even die when they are supposed to. Then you can get too many of them in your blood and they don't work right. When some of your white blood cells are sick, the healthy white blood cells can't do their job well. This is called leukemia.

♥ **Platelets** are tiny bits of cells that act like little stoppers that plug up leaks caused by holes. That keeps you from bleeding, because they form blood clots. You want to have just the right amount of platelets so that they can fill up the holes and keep your blood where it is supposed to be. When they are low, you get nosebleeds and have bleeding elsewhere, too.

Now that you know a little about how your blood works, you can follow along with how Kevin used this information to send good messages to his blood. Kevin feels so powerful now when he talks to his white blood cells. He feels stronger inside with his white blood cells listening to him.

Tap along with us so your white blood cells can feel good too.

ROUND 1

White Blood Cells

Tap on the Karate Chop point and say:

Even though part of my blood got sick, I'm a great kid.

Even though my white blood cells don't feel well, I'm a great kid.

Even though my body is sick, I love myself.

Eyebrow: I have sick white blood cells.

Side of the Eye: They call it leukemia.

Under the Eye: My blood cells are not healthy.

Under the Nose: My white blood cells are in bad shape.

Chin: They are not healthy. They are sick.

Collarbone: They aren't working right.

Under the Arm: They don't do their job right.

Top of the Head: Right now, my blood is not healthy and neither am I.

ROUND 2

Eyebrow: I know my white blood cells are doing the best they can, while not feeling well.

Side of the Eye: I know they are trying to defend me even when they are sick.

Under the Eye: I know they are doing the best they can.

Under the Nose: I appreciate that they keep trying to do their best.

Chin: It is difficult for my white blood cells to work right when they are not healthy.

Collarbone: And when I'm feeling negative it's even worse for us both. I would like them to get better so they can work right to defend me.

Under the Arm: I love my white blood cells, even though they are in bad shape right now.

Top of the Head: I love my white blood cells, even though they are sick.

ROUND 3

Eyebrow: I can talk to my white blood cells. Yes, I can do that.

Side of the Eye: I'm allowed to talk to my white blood cells.

Under the Eye: I think of them as little kids who want lots of love and attention.

Under the Nose: I give them love and attention.

Chin: I tell them I know they don't feel good.

Collarbone: I tell them that they are loved anyway. They didn't do anything wrong.

Under the Arm: They can get better now and so can I.

Top of the Head: It is okay for us to get better together. I want to get better.

ROUND 4

Eyebrow: I know they are listening to me.

Side of the Eye: I want them to hear good thoughts from me.

Under the Eye: I want them to know how much I appreciate them and how much I want to get better.

Chin: I'm going to tell them happy and fun things every day.

Collarbone: I am going to tell them how wonderful they are.

Under the Nose: I tell them I want them to be strong and good defenders. I tell them they are incredibly special — just like me.

Top of the Head: I want to feel good and I want my white blood cells to feel good, too.

ROUND 5

Eyebrow: I don't know what happened to make my blood cells not work right.

Side of the Eye: But that doesn't matter, because I talk to them every day about getting better.

Under the Eye: I know that my cells are listening to me, so I tell them what I want them to hear.

Under the Nose: I tell them how much I love them, how much I appreciate them and how much I want them to fix themselves and get better.

Chin: I keep sending the message that I want them to fix themselves.

Collarbone: My body is really smart and it knows how to fix itself.

Under the Arm: I want my body to have everything it needs to fix itself.

Top of the Head: I trust that my body can fix itself.

ROUND 6

Eyebrow: I'm going to do my part.

Side of the Eye: I'm going to send good messages to my cells every day.

Under the Eye: I'm going to send them happy thoughts.

Under the Nose: I send them laughter and smiles.

Chin: I send them lots of love, too.

Collarbone: I send them happy messages and thank them for all their work.

Under the Arm: I tell them how good they are.

Top of the Head: Just like I'm a good kid.

ROUND 7 — RED BLOOD CELLS

Eyebrow: My red blood cells love picking up oxygen and taking it all over my body.

Side of the Eye: I remember to breathe deeply to help them do this.

Under the Eye: I take deep breaths and my red blood cells say, "Yeah! More oxygen!"

Under the Nose: They gladly pick it up and carry it to the parts of my body that need it. They are very smart.

Chin: That oxygen makes me feel alive.

Collarbone: My red blood cells love carrying oxygen throughout my body.

Under the Arm: They drop it off where it is needed and take the waste out.

Top of the Head: I breathe deeply to help them out and I feel more alive.

ROUND 8 — PLATELETS

Eyebrow: My platelets are great.

Side of the Eye: They are the greatest little stoppers in the world.

Under the Eye: They plug up any holes that would let me bleed.

Under the Nose: I love that they know exactly how to do their job.

Chin: I ask my body to make just the right number of platelets.

Collarbone: Just enough to stop any bleeding.

Under the Arm: Not too many, not too few. Just the right number.

Top of the Head: My platelets help me get better and I thank them.

ROUND 9 — ALL THREE TOGETHER

Eyebrow: My defenses are made up of my white blood cells.

Side of the Eye: They are helped by my red blood cells and platelets.

Under the Eye: I like that I have a whole team of cells that work together to help me get better.

Under the Nose: I love that they defend me and do their best to make me healthy.

Chin: I love that my defenses are really intelligent.

Collarbone: My defenses help out so that my cells can fix themselves.

Under the Arm: They know exactly how to repair themselves.

Top of the Head: I'd like them to repair themselves.

ROUND 10

Eyebrow: All my cells work well together. In fact, they work perfectly! Like a perfect harmony.

Side of the Eye: My red blood cells, my white blood cells and platelets are all working together in harmony.

Under the Eye: They are a team and they help me be healthy.

Under the Nose: I love that my red and white blood cells and platelets work together as a team.

Chin: They are a great team to help all my cells get healthy and stay healthy.

Collarbone: And they have such a good time helping each other out.

Under the Arm: I love helping them, too — by being happy!

Top of the Head: I help them out by sending them good thoughts and lots of love. Whoo hoo!!

ROUND 11

Eyebrow: I'm so proud of them, because they help me get healthy and stay healthy.

Side of the Eye: I'm going to do my part too. I'm going to be part of the team.

Under the Eye: I'm going to be positive and happy, so they can be even stronger.

Under the Nose: Together we are going to beat this problem.

Chin: Together we are going to defend ourselves.

Collarbone: Together we are even stronger than if we were working alone.

Under the Arm: Together we are quite an amazing force — a force of power and strength.

Top of the Head: Together we get stronger and more powerful — and we build strong blood cells and a strong body.

ROUND 12

Eyebrow: I never used to talk to my white blood cells, but now I do.

Side of the Eye: I love my white blood cells and tell them so every day.

Under the Eye: I know they need to hear how much they are loved.

Under the Nose: I send my white blood cells light and love.

Chin: I send them hugs and kisses.

Collarbone: I know they want to get better. I give them permission to get better.

Under the Arm: I want my white blood cells to get better.

Top of the Head: If we work together, we can get better together. Anything is possible if we work together!

ROUND 13

Eyebrow: I imagine my white blood cells surrounded by love — red love. (You can choose a different color if you like — whatever color you feel love is.)

Side of the Eye: I surround each and every white blood cell with loving RED.

Under the Eye: I bathe my white blood cells in red love.

Under the Nose: I don't get mad at them for being sick. I love them instead.

Chin: I know they feel awful and want lots of love. Just like me when I feel sick.

Collarbone: I send them lots and lots of love — red love. I send them red love because they are wonderful, just like me.

Under the Arm: The more love I send them, the better they feel.

Top of the Head: I surround them with lots and lots of beautiful red love.

ROUND 14

Eyebrow: I send my red blood cells love.

Side of the Eye: I send my white blood cells love.

Under the Eye: I send my platelets love.

Chin: I send love to my whole defense team.

Collarbone: I send love to all of my cells.

Under the Arm: I especially send love to the parts of my body that don't feel good.

Top of the Head: What a great team – a great defense team – all working together to make me healthy.

Kevin feels so much better now because he is paying attention to what he thinks and feels. By being positive he is helping his body get a message that will help it feel better too. Now *that* is powerful.

Keep telling your white blood cells just how much you love them. Keep sending them red love, too (or whatever color you have chosen). Just like a little kid, they want to be reminded how much you love them and how much you want them to work well. Send love to your red blood cells and platelets, too.

It is also important to send love and kind thoughts to the rest of your body. It will help your body work wonderfully and feel stronger and happier. Sending love to your body puts you in control of what you feel and that makes you powerful. And when you are powerful, incredible things happen.

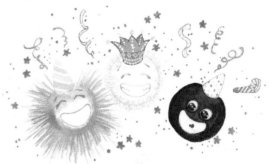

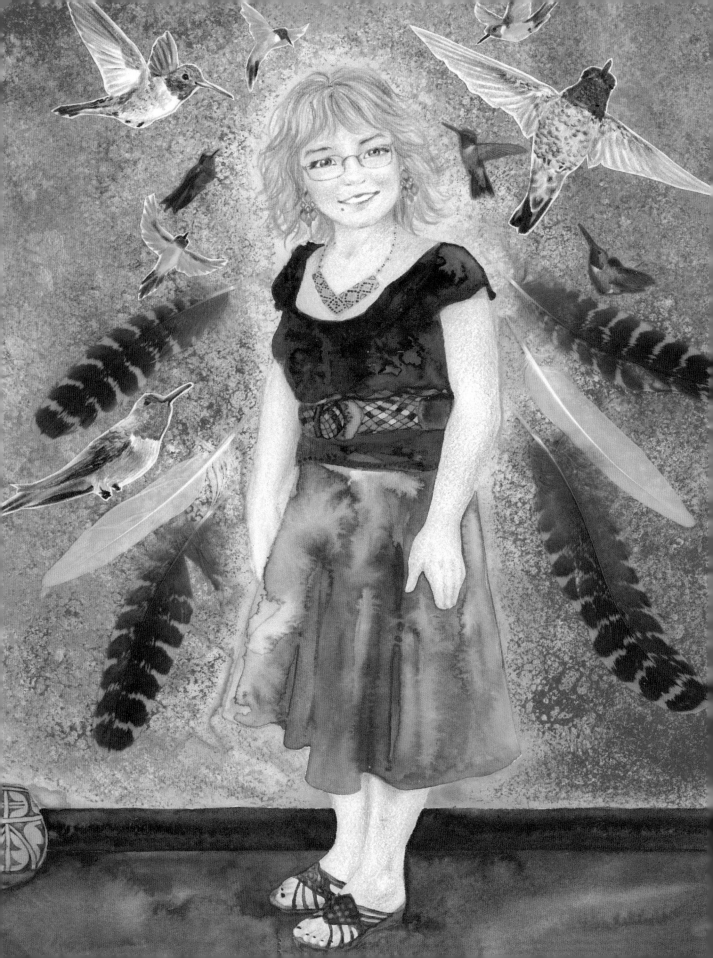

CONCLUSION

*F*rom my personal experiences working with so many children with serious illness, I know that managing one's emotions can have a huge impact on how a child deals with treatments. Ultimately, this changes the whole process and experience, as well as the outcome. No matter what happens, if a child feels loved, cared for and empowered, then a true gift has been given to them. If they feel that they can play an active role in their own recovery and can consciously choose to feel joy and happiness rather than pain and suffering, this gives them back a sense of hope. Although it may not be easy to calculate the effects of this, it is clear that feeling hopeful, positive and calm is vital to any recovery process.

One's body begins to make changes for the better, too. Family relations also improve with the help of EFT or Tapping, and become enriched by the recovery process, rather than being damaged or torn apart by the stress of it.

In the stories in this book, I have teamed Tapping together with voicing any desired physical changes. This is a powerful combination, as it works on many different levels. Consequently, it can have a profound impact on how the body heals.

Having your child take an active part in this process is key. He or she will have an idea of how the body heals and get to see how their words, thoughts and feelings affect what's happening within their bodies. They become active participants in their healing process. What a powerful tool in their hands!

Epigenetics is the link between the mind and genetics. According to Bruce Lipton, Ph.D., when you change your behavior, you are also reprogramming your genetics. Thus, Epigenetics shows that the body responds to how one thinks, feels and to what one experiences — even to what one eats. These are all messages being sent into our body's cells, which then respond by producing the substances the body needs to respond appropriately to those incoming messages.

Sending a positive message to the body allows it to respond in a way that creates healing substances. Remember to be persistent and have faith. Continuity in the positive messages we send to our cells is important. It helps the 'get better' messages to enter the body effectively. This sort of 'well-wishing' supports the immune system and helps it to take care of the body.

My heartfelt desire is that this book will be of service to you. I hope that it helps and supports you in this journey. May you find that the techniques within this book inspire you to be in charge of your own life, emotions and the outcomes of them, thereby improving the quality of your life experience and that of your children on a daily basis. Most importantly, may the stories recounted here fill your heart with love. Thank you for reading them.

DEBORAH'S INSPIRED GOAL AND HOW YOU CAN BE PART OF IT

I am dedicating myself to helping at least one million of you —men, women and children — to prevent future illness (mental, emotional or physical) using the simplest, easiest and most economical methods. I want you to be happy, healthy and prosperous. My goal is to empower you to have the ability to release your fears, anxieties, past traumas and childhood beliefs and patterns that hold you back while subsequently building your self-confidence and self-love. In addition, I'm passionate about teaching you to use these accessible methods that empower a person to make wise decisions that allow the body to regenerate and restore itself, emotionally and physically.

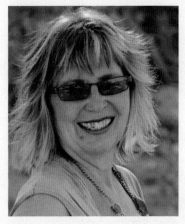

ABOUT THE AUTHOR

Deborah D. Miller has her Ph.D. degree in Cell and Molecular Biology, and is currently living in Oaxaca, Mexico. She is passionate about helping people release the emotional charges and traumas of their lives, especially the ones from childhood. She skillfully does this using her scientific mind and her intuition.

Deborah is an EFT Expert and Trainer, certified by the founder of EFT (Gary Craig), AAMET and the Spanish EFT Association (AHEFT). She is a Deeksha Giver, Reiki Master, Nutritional Guide and Personal Motivation Guide. She understands the necessity of working with the emotional aspects underlying 'dis-ease' within the body and the need to cleanse and nourish the physical body. Her personal journey of improving her own immune system gives her hands-on experience of the requirements for improving one's energy levels and health.

Deborah began volunteering in the children's cancer wing of Hospital General Aurelio Validivieso in Oaxaca, Mexico, in September of 2007. She applied EFT and other energy techniques to the children, parents and nurses to help them reduce stress, fear and anxiety and improve their mental and emotional health. She does this work in a way that is complementary to the treatments given by the hospital. Helping these children have tools to manage their emotions has led to a heart-felt passion to help more and more children all over the world.

FOR FURTHER CONTACT, CONSULTATION AND INFORMATION

Deborah D. Miller, Ph.D.
www.FindTheLightWithin.com
www.OaxacaProject.com
ddmiller7@FindTheLightWithin.com
713 893 3440 US
951 515 3332 Mexico

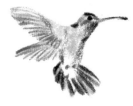

SOME THINGS YOU CAN DO

♥ Tap every day.

♥ Work with a trained EFT practitioner to release your main emotional issues.

♥ Tap with your children playfully.

♥ Share the power of EFT Tapping:
  – tell friends what it's done for you!
  – show them how to tap.
  – send them to an EFT practitioner.
  – keep Tapping regularly. The extraordinary benefits will affect not only you, but also those around you!

♥ Organize Tapping Parties! Gather a group of people who want to tap together – perhaps to lose weight, or address stress. Or just gather to tap on positive phrases for fun and well-being!

♥ Feel free to contact me to lead your first Tapping Party, or instruct a group you have organized to use EFT for serious illness.

♥ Subscribe to my newsletter at www.FindTheLightWithin.com.

♥ Donate this book to a family in need, or to the children's area of a hospital.

♥ Donate EFT Tapping sessions with a professional to a child with cancer.

♥ If you are an EFT practitioner, donate your Tapping services to a family in need.

♥ Do other health supporting activities to improve your family's nutrition and strengthen the immune system. Sign up for my classes, "Fermented Vegetables" and "Green Drinks." Tap, Eat & Drink your way to health!

JOIN IN TO CREATE A WORLDWIDE EFT TAPPING COMMUNITY!

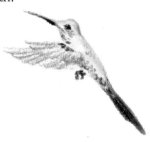

REFERENCES

Church, D. (2013). Clinical EFT as an Evidence-Based Practice for the Treatment of Psychological and Physiological Conditions. *Psychology*, 4(8).

Church, D., Hawk, C., Brooks, A.J., Toukolehto, O., Wren, M., Dinter, I., & Stein, P. (2013). Psychological Trauma Symptom Improvement in Veterans Using Emotional Freedom Techniques. *Journal of Nervous and Mental Disease,* 201(2), 153-160.

Church, D., & Books, A. (2010). Application of Emotional Freedom Techniques. *Integrative Medicine: A Clinician's Journal*, Aug/Sep, 46-48.

Church, D., Geronilla, L., & Dinter, I. (2009). Psychological symptom change in veterans after six sessions of Emotional Freedom Techniques (EFT): An observational study. [Electronic journal article]. *International Journal of Healing and Caring, 9*(1).

Church, D., Yount, G., & Brooks, A. (2012). The Effect of Emotional Freedom Techniques (EFT) on Stress Biochemistry: A Randomized Controlled Trial. *Journal of Nervous and Mental Disease*, Oct. 200(10), 891-6.

Feinstein, D. (2012). Acupoint stimulation in treating psychological disorders: Evidence of efficacy. *Review of General Psychology*, 16, 364-380.

Feinstein, D. (2010). Rapid Treatment of PTSD: Why Psychological Exposure with Acupoint Tapping May Be Effective. *Psychotherapy: Theory, Research, Practice, Training*, 47(3), 385-402.

Feinstein, D. (2008). Energy Psychology: A Review of the Preliminary Evidence. *Psychotherapy: Theory, Research, Practice, Training*, 45(2), 199-213.

Feinstein, D. (2008). Energy Psychology in Disaster Relief. *Traumatology*, 14, 124-137.

Feinstein, D., & Eden, D. (2008). Six pillars of energy medicine: Clinical strengths of a complementary paradigm. *Alternative Therapies*, 14(1), 44-54.

Gruder, D. (2012). Controversial 2008 Research Review Published in Psychotherapy Finds New Support. *Psychotherapy Bulletin. Official Publication of Division 29 of the American Psychological Association*, Volume 47, Number 3.

Lipton, B. (2008). *The Biology of Belief: Unleashing the Power of Consciousness, Matter & Miracles.* Original Copyright © 2005 by Bruce Lipton. Revised copyright © 2008 by Mountain of Love Productions. Published by Hay House, Inc.

Moore, K.L., & Agur, A.M. (2007). *Essential Clinical Anatomy: Third Edition.* Baltimore: Lippincott Williams & Wilkins 42.

Waitem W., & Holder, M. (2003). Assessment of the Emotional Freedom Technique: An Alternative Treatment for Fear. *The Scientific Review of Mental Health Practice*, (2)1.

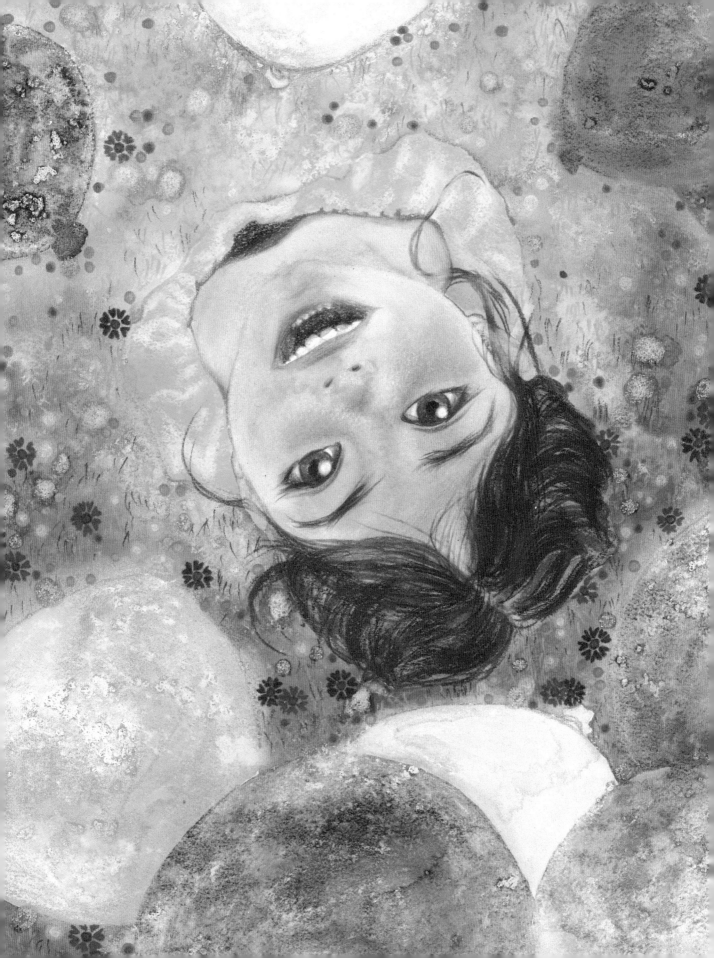